# SWEET DREAMS

## *A Comprehensive Guide to Guaranteed Baby Sleep*

**By**
**Lindsey Kohn, M.S, MFT**

# Table of Contents

# Introduction

Are you a new mom worried about getting your baby to sleep? Or maybe you've been through this before and don't want to deal with sleepless nights again.

Babies don't have regular sleep patterns, and they're prevalent. But knowing the tactics for putting them to sleep is a special skill that a mother can have. According to the pediatrician, Dr. Reshmi Bashu, newborns sleep longer, but as they grow older, their need for sleep decreases, as cited in Children's Health of Orange County (2021). They sleep up to 16 hours during a 24-hour period but intermittently, meaning they wake up every 2–3 hours depending on the reason—they either wake up because they're hungry, their diaper needs a change, or they need a cuddle from their mother.

Parents with newborns experience challenges and show a range of emotions—good and bad. They are adjusting to these challenges through their response mechanisms. However, what's alarming is when they're too exhausted, seeking the need for sleep because they can't function well throughout the day and lack the focus they need for work and running a household. Imagine you're alone with your newborn, who cries now and then and does not even sleep for an hour or two. You can't even sleep for 7–8 hours straight, as recommended by Miller (2017). If you are deprived of sleep, you are more likely to suffer from mood and postpartum sleep disorders, which are leading risk factors for depression.

Consider the experience of Elaine Jacobson, shared by Dr. Patricia Santiago-Munoz (2015), to highlight the challenges she faced. At 18, Elaine became pregnant and couldn't pursue higher education. Dealing with hearing loss compounded her struggles, leaving her feeling worthless as she couldn't breastfeed her baby due to stress. Though she eventually coped, 11 years later, she became pregnant again. This time was different; she neglected her wellbeing, experiencing paranoia and disconnect. Doubts crept in, questioning the decision to have another child. Seeking professional help, she learned that her mood swings were not just baby blues but postpartum depression. Through prescribed medications, she found relief and improved her situation.

Parenthood is tough—especially for new mothers—and if they couldn't bear it, they might end up getting stressed—postpartum depression, so to speak. This depression comes with a feeling of worthlessness, anger, irritability, other mood swings, and worst of all, suicide (Mayo Clinic, 2022).

Moreover, disregarding sleep deprivation could result in unfavorable outcomes for both children and parents. In a study by Richter et al. (2019), focusing on new parents, it was found that sleep satisfaction and duration notably decreased after childbirth, especially affecting women within the initial three months. It took approximately six years for sleep contentment and duration to recover.

Sleep is crucial for the mother's emotional wellbeing, which will eventually lead to holistic health in the long run. Parents who are stressed will pass it on to their babies, and they'll respond to it by demonstrating physiological changes (Dallas Sleep, n.d.). So, when you are sleep deprived, you are more likely to endanger your child's safety. This is because you are more prone to slips and mishaps, which you don't want to happen when holding your baby.

A common practice among mothers is taking a nap while their babies sleep. Due to household chores that need to be finished while babies are slumbering, this practice can be challenging, but quick power naps of 10–20 minutes can provide rejuvenation. With sufficient rest, you can manage various tasks, such as preparing nutritious meals and handling laundry. Acquiring the skill to put your baby to sleep offers wholesome advantages for you, your spouse, and the entire family, fostering a joyful household imbued with affection and warmth.

You're not alone on your parenting journey. If many have survived, why wouldn't you? Preparation and being knowledgeable about taking good care of your baby and—of course—yourself may result in happier parenting. Alongside your loved ones, who are ready to help you along the way, your inspiration (which is your baby or kids), and a well-conditioned mind, you will get through it, and your baby will be happy as they grow with you!

But if your child's sleep problems are interfering with your own, the best thing you can do is train them to sleep better. It offers your baby pride and independence to self-soothe and go to sleep on their own. And it will provide you with much-needed relaxation as well as sleep. But the question is: *How*?

# Chapter 1: Understanding Baby Sleep

It's important for parents to have knowledge about baby sleep to ensure their little ones get adequate rest as they grow. Newborns do not have a clear day-night schedule, so they sleep whenever they feel like it. It's beneficial if they sleep more at night, but what if they want to be awake and active? Babies require a lot of sleep, but their small tummies need frequent feeding, even during the night. Understanding these sleep patterns is crucial for planning your next steps.

## *Sleep Cycles at Different Stages*

Babies and toddlers require varying amounts of sleep, depending on their age. Newborns (0–3 months) typically sleep for approximately 14–17 hours, while infants (4–11 months) generally sleep for about 12–15 hours. Toddlers (1–2 years) typically get around 11–14 hours of sleep, and preschoolers (3–5 years) need about 10–13 hours. The need for ample sleep is evident due to their high level of activity during the day (National Sleep Foundation, 2015).

Even though these sleep ranges might be surprising, you may still struggle to sleep for long stretches. Babies sleep in cycles of about 50–60 minutes, and they wake up crying when they're hungry or need a change. For instance, newborns cry often in their first three months because they need you for feeding, diaper changes, and comfort.

Raising Children Network (RCN) says babies need sleep to grow and develop well. But their sleep needs are different from those of older kids. Some babies might need more or less sleep than others their age.

Babies' wellbeing and mood are like signals that show if they're getting enough sleep.

- If your baby is happy and alert, they're getting enough sleep.

- If your baby is fussy, they need more sleep.

When babies sleep, they move around a lot, twitching their arms and legs, smiling, and even sucking. They use different ways to show they need sleep, like crying, rubbing their eyes, or fussing.

From 2 to 12 months old, babies' sleep changes a lot. They might sleep more at night and less during the day. They stay awake for longer between naps. So, they need less sleep at night and might wake up less, which is good news for parents!

At 2–3 months, babies sleep on and off all day and night. They have sleep cycles that last about 50–60 minutes. Each cycle includes active and quiet sleep. In active sleep, babies move and grunt, but in quiet sleep, they're still. They wake up at the end of each cycle, and they might cry or make noises. They might need help settling back to sleep. Also, they might start sleeping more at night.

From 3 to 6 months, they sleep on and off for about 12–15 hours a day. They might take 2–3 shorter naps in the afternoon. Nights become longer, and some might sleep around six hours at a time by six months. You can tell if they're in deep sleep if they're still, or in light sleep if they wake up easily. You'll get to know more about active and quiet sleep later.

Between 6 and 12 months, most babies are ready for bed between 6 and 10 p.m. They usually fall asleep in less than 40 minutes. Their sleep is more like adults', so they might wake up less at night. But many still wake up and need help going back to sleep. Some might do this 3–4 times each night.

As babies get older, they sleep less and take 2–3 naps during the day, each lasting 30 minutes to 2 hours. By the time they're one year old, they'll probably sleep around 11–14 hours each day. At six months, they learn new things that might disrupt their sleep, like these examples (RCN, n.d.):

- Babies start to understand things and know you exist. So, if you leave the room, they might cry for you.

- When babies start crawling, they might have trouble settling down to sleep. Moving more can change how they sleep.

- Babies learn to stay awake, especially when exciting things are happening around them, like noise and light.

- Babies can get upset when their moms aren't around. This might make them not want to sleep and wake up a lot at night. But as they grow, they get better at handling this fear.

When babies are put to bed feeling sleepy but still awake, they learn to soothe themselves. This helps them fall asleep on their own at bedtime and go back to sleep if they wake up during the night. On another note, babies who always rely on their parents to fall asleep might become used to calling out for help in the middle of the night.

Other things can affect babies' sleep too. Babies who feel close and secure with their caregiver might have fewer sleep problems. But some babies might find it hard to sleep without being held. Babies might also start feeling anxious when they're away from their parents in the second half of the year. Sickness and learning to move around a lot quickly can also make it harder for babies to sleep well.

When babies turn one to two years old, hence the term toddlers, they need about 11 to 14 hours of sleep each day. They usually take naps starting around 18 months old, and these naps become shorter, lasting one to three hours. It's a good idea for toddlers to have their nap a bit earlier in the day, so it doesn't affect their nighttime sleep.

Toddlers often have sleep troubles. They might have a tough time falling asleep or wake up a lot at night. Nightmares and being scared of the dark are common too. Many things can cause these sleep issues, like wanting to be independent and working on new thinking, social, and movement skills. These changes can make it tricky for toddlers to settle down and sleep well.

## *Science Behind Sleep Cycles*

Have you ever gone through this? You've given your baby a bath, made her all comfy with powder, set up the crib, and rocked her to sleep while feeding. Everything seemed perfect, and your baby fell asleep. But just when you thought you could relax, your baby starts crying and wants you to help her sleep again. This cycle keeps repeating, and it feels like it will never stop. Does this ring a bell with you?

Well, it's common with newborns—but like I said earlier, if you know how to put your baby to sleep without those intervals of waking up, you have that special skill as a mother. In addition, knowing the science behind these sleep cycles would also help you understand your baby's development.

It makes sense that many parents want their babies to sleep through the night. The more peacefully a baby sleeps, the more soundly their parents may rest. Sadly, parents must understand that their babies will wake up numerous times throughout the night because they lack a strong circadian rhythm that causes others—adults and older children—to feel weary at night instead of during the day (Pacheco, 2023). No wonder newborns wake up frequently at night.

*The body's internal clock is naturally aligned with the cycle of day and night.* –Eric Suni

The body operates on 24-hour cycles known as *circadian rhythms,* which drive essential functions and processes (Suni, 2020). Among these rhythms, the sleep-wake cycle is particularly well-known and significant. Coordinated by the brain's biological clock, circadian rhythms are synchronized across various bodily systems. These rhythms are intertwined with the day-night cycle, heavily influenced by external cues like light.

When correctly aligned, a circadian rhythm supports regular and rejuvenating sleep. Speaking of rejuvenating sleep in babies, it refers to an uninterrupted, undisturbed night's sleep, commonly known as sleeping through the night (West, 2015). However, if this circadian cycle is disrupted, it can lead to severe sleep problems like insomnia. As babies are still adapting to the external world, they haven't yet established a synchronized circadian rhythm. With time, they'll grasp the concept that nights are meant for rest, not play.

Between three months and a year of age, most babies start adopting a sleep routine more akin to that of adults. They tend to nap briefly during the day and experience longer sleep periods at night (Pacheco, 2023). Yet not all infants adhere to an adult-like sleep schedule at the same age. If your one-year-old isn't sleeping through the night, don't be alarmed. Many babies continue to wake up at least once a night even beyond the first year.

Researchers explain that infants older than three months have four sleep stages, compared to the two stages in newborns, as noted by Pacheco (2023). These stages encompass non-rapid eye movement (NREM) and rapid eye movement (REM) sleep. The NREM is known as quiet sleep, while the REM is active sleep. Babies exhibit bodily movements during active sleep, or REM, including jaw and eye movements, finger and limb twitches. In contrast, during quiet sleep, or NREM, they remain still.

Around three months of age, babies begin experiencing the same sleep stages as adults. These four stages comprise three NREM stages and one REM stage. Distinguished by brain wave patterns, these stages are described as follows (Felson, 2005):

- Stage 1: Drifting off (NREM); the eyes are closed but easily awakened.

- Stage 2: Light sleep (NREM); the body prepares for deep sleep.

- Stage 3: Deep sleep (NREM); waking can become more challenging, potentially resulting in confusion if one is abruptly awakened.

- Stage 4: Dream sleep (REM); the brain is more active during the dreaming phase.

Felson (2005) reveals that babies spend 50% of their sleep time in REM, while adults spend 20%. This equates to around nine REM episodes in 24 hours due to babies' extended sleep.

Although babies start experiencing the four sleep stages around three months, it isn't until closer to five months that their sleep patterns, including time spent in each stage, resemble those of adults (Pacheco, 2023). Remarkably, babies enter REM shortly after falling asleep, unlike adults, who experience REM sleep after about 90 minutes.

In newborns, sleep cycles involve two stages: active and quiet sleep. Over time, these patterns evolve, with less time spent in REM sleep. As babies grow, they encounter NREM sleep in three stages rather than just one. Eventually, their sleep patterns become more adult-like.

These sleep cycles repeat during both long naps and nighttime sleep. Babies typically experience sleep cycles of about 40 minutes, leading to more frequent awakenings.

## *Factors Affecting Baby Sleep*

A combination of environmental and genetic factors can impact a baby's sleep patterns (Dewar, 2018). For instance, hereditary factors might explain nearly half of the individual variations in nighttime sleep duration (Dewar, 2018). Conversely, individual differences in napping patterns are mostly influenced by environmental factors, such as whether parents encourage napping.

How do genes affect a baby's sleep habits? One way is by influencing a baby's disposition or temperament. Babies who are less adaptable and fussier tend to be more challenging to soothe. Furthermore, research suggests that such babies tend to sleep less on average (Dewar, 2018).

It's possible that some babies naturally require less sleep than others, and genes contribute to specific aspects of how babies sleep, like how easily and quickly they can be roused. Nonetheless, it's undeniable that parents can influence their baby's sleep habits. They can incorporate the circadian cycle into their baby's routine and help them learn to self-soothe back to sleep when they wake up at night.

Baby sleep habits vary from one country to another. Studies reveal that babies in Italy and Japan often sleep less than babies in Switzerland and Canada (Dewar, 2018). It's very likely that how babies sleep, what's considered normal, and what they need could be different in various parts of the world due to factors like time, history, location, culture, and society (Abbott, 2021).

Conversely, achieving motor milestones like walking, standing, or crawling can frequently disrupt a baby's sleep cycle. Until around six months of age, most babies won't have developed the ability to self-soothe or sleep through the night. The first key point to remember is that timing is crucial. Creating a routine for bedtimes, nap times, and wake-up times can greatly benefit your child by ensuring they get the right amount and quality of sleep.

One of the most challenging aspects of parenting is ensuring that both your children and yourself get adequate and restful sleep. However, it's important to put effort into mastering this skill. By becoming attuned to your baby's sleep patterns and cycles and learning to interpret their cues, you can make small adjustments that enhance the wellbeing of your entire family.

# Chapter 2:
# Creating a Sleep-Conducive Environment

Lights off! That's the universal signal for bedtime. Just like you, newborns and children also associate darkness with sleep. A softly lit room with minimal noise translates to a quieter environment for your baby. This reduced stimulation cues their young minds that it's time to settle down. Maintaining a consistent level of darkness once your child is in bed can contribute to improved sleep quality. Imagine that someone flips on the lights while you're sleeping; you get disturbed. Now imagine how much more impactful it is for babies.

However, creating the right sleep environment involves more than just adjusting the lighting. There are other factors to consider when establishing a conducive atmosphere for your little one.

## Designing a Calming Nursery

Just like our cozy home—a haven of tranquility—the nursery should also exude a calming and visually pleasing atmosphere. It shouldn't be cluttered or have a chaotic interior design. The last thing you want is for the nursery to be distracting and unwelcoming, especially for your baby. So, how can you create a soothing and inviting space? Willes (2017), the author of *Getting Your Baby to Sleep: The Baby Sleep Trainer Way*, emphasizes that whether you're room-sharing with your baby or not, there are four key elements to consider:

Firstly, minimize natural and artificial lighting. The room should be as dark as possible, not just during the night but also for every nap. Light from various sources—bulbs, lamps, or windows—can disrupt the circadian rhythms. When there's light, your body signals that it's not time to rest, and babies respond the same way. Some parents struggle to put their newborns to sleep at night, not realizing that proper training and an appropriately designed nursery play crucial roles. The room should be so dark that you can't read the words in a book anymore. This darkness is conducive to your newborn's sound sleep, so consider using thick curtains to block out sunlight. If even small lights manage to sneak in from the sides of the curtains, use hook-and-loop tape to ensure they're firmly in place, creating a pitch-dark environment.

If you need to enter the room, ensure the hallway light is off to avoid introducing bright light. And if you need some light for changing diapers or feeding, a 15-watt light bulb is sufficient for baby-related tasks. Don't worry about potentially disrupting their long-term sleep pattern. Keeping the room dark won't confuse them about day and night. This phenomenon is common among newborns and typically resolves itself after a few weeks. For nighttime tasks, consider using a dim red bulb, as red light has the least negative impact.

Secondly, avoid stuffed animals or objects that make noise at intervals, as well as items that create detectable loops or beats. While these may contribute to an aesthetically pleasing nursery, they are only beneficial when your baby is awake or a bit older. Instead, opt for a white noise machine that mimics a fan-like sound, or position an electric fan in a way that promotes restorative sleep for your baby. A study in 1990 (Spencer et al.) on newborn sleep and white noise found that 80% of the 40 newborns fell asleep within 5 minutes using a white noise machine, compared to 25% without it. Another study (Sezici & Yigit, 2017) showed that babies fell asleep more easily and cried less with white noise, compared to those soothed in a swing. According to the American Academy of Pediatrics (2016), playing white noise at a low volume can help babies relax, as the humming, muffled sound reminds them of their time in the womb.

Thirdly, use baby monitors, but place them away from the crib. Some parents place cameras inside the crib for a clear view of their baby's movements, but this is not advisable, as anything inside the crib could potentially harm the baby. It's best to mount the monitor on the wall. The same rule applies to white noise machines—ensure they are out of the baby's reach. Baby monitors provide peace of mind by allowing you to keep an eye on your baby even when you're not in the same room. They offer reassurance and help alleviate constant anxiety. What makes monitors soothing for babies is their two-way communication feature. You can interact with your baby even from another room, making it easier to comfort them until you arrive.

Lastly, invest in a sturdy, safe crib. A safe crib means a mattress without elevation or incline, a snug-fitting sheet, and a robust mesh bumper. The sleep environment, including the crib or bed style, mattress quality, and other factors, plays a pivotal role in fostering healthy sleeping patterns for your child. A single stuffed toy and a pacifier can also provide additional comfort, but ensure the toy is 12 inches square or smaller and withdraw the pacifier before they reach 12 months. According to Decker (2022), frequent pacifier use or vigorous thumb sucking can lead to dental issues. Try not to rely on the pacifier excessively. If your baby continues to cry while in the crib, it might be due to a dirty mattress or other factors. It's wise to thoroughly check everything in the crib, as dust mites, bugs, ants, and other small insects could be interfering with your baby's sleep and comfort. To maintain a hygienic crib, deep clean the mattress every month and wash the bedding weekly.

Parents strive to prevent their babies from suffering during this phase—it's a double win that leads to a positive outcome. To ease the burden, adhering to these four elements for a comfortable sleeping environment for your baby, along with maintaining your sanity, can make a significant difference. After all, the wellbeing of your children is of the utmost importance.

## Controlling Lighting and Temperature

Since lighting affects sleep, it's crucial to delve deeper into this topic, as it provides a soothing glow throughout the room for your baby. Opting for a room with windows can be beneficial, as natural light and fresh air are preferable to artificial alternatives, especially when the weather is favorable. However, when it comes to sleeping during inclement weather, you need to be intentional about the type of lighting and temperature required for that specific situation.

### Natural Lighting

Do you have a baby who seems to be hosting a party at 3 a.m.? This likely indicates that their circadian rhythms are still not synchronized. The internal clock's rhythm is significantly influenced by natural light. Exposure to this light is the most effective way to help your baby recognize that it's time to be awake and not time to sleep.

Natural light not only enhances human performance but also helps balance circadian rhythms. For babies, it plays a critical role in helping them adjust to a regular 24-hour day. However, it takes time for circadian rhythms, which control the sleep-wake cycle and contribute to newborns' irregular sleep patterns, to fully develop. This usually occurs around six weeks of age (National Sleep Foundation, 2015).

To ensure that your baby receives the necessary quality sleep for their development, it's essential for parents to aid their bodies in establishing healthy sleep patterns.

### Ceiling-Mounted, Ambient Lighting

The main source of light in a room is called ambient lighting, otherwise known as general lighting. You don't want a bright, harsh one since it'll entirely ruin the room's ambience, and worse, your baby's comfort. Consider a ceiling-mounted fixture, as it may facilitate quiet wind-down activities, reading, and midnight changes or feeds. Because this is your baby's bedroom, you don't want to disturb them while they're sleeping, so pick lights with a warm color temperature, e.g., 4400°F, to create a calm and tranquil environment.

Avoid using exposed bulbs and halogens. These intense lights make babies uneasy and anxious, and they may even be dangerous if they are curious about them. Instead, choose lighting fixtures that provide diffused or veiled light. For a baby's eyes, daylight and soft white bulbs are preferable.

Even the University of Notre Dame (n.d.) recommends ambient lighting as the standard source of light in the Newborn Intensive Care Unit (NICU), that is, having 10–600 lumens, a measurement for appropriate room brightness. Both natural and electric lighting also have settings that provide quick darkness in any bed position to enable transillumination. So, you can conclude that ambient lighting is more advisable.

### Nighttime Lighting

The controversy between vision and baby night lights started in the study of Quinn et al. (1999), published in the journal *Nature*. Researchers discovered a link between ambient night light and myopia, or nearsightedness. But only survey data was used to draw this association, not their medical examination or records. They didn't take genetics into account, which could have had a greater impact on their vision. Nonetheless, a study by Chapell et al. (2001) published in *Perceptual & Motor Skills*, which was contrary to the prior one, concluded that myopia and night lights do not correlate in children 0–2 years of age who slept in darkness with hall lights, room lights, and night lights.

Now, the American Optometric Association (n.d.) recommends parents leave a nightlight or dim light on in their baby's nursery to support visual development, especially from birth to four months. Also, night lights are useful to keep the lighting dim while changing diapers and feeding babies at night.

### Task Lighting

It's late at night, and your baby is calling out for you. You enter the room but hesitate to turn on the lights, fearing it might disrupt your baby's sleep. To address this, consider using a task light, like a dim lamp, which provides gentle illumination for nighttime feeding or diaper changes without being harsh on both you and the baby. While rocking your baby to sleep, you can use the lamp until they fall asleep again.

Task lighting adds extra light to specific areas in a room that might already be somewhat lit. If you prefer softer lighting, go for adjustable table lamps (avoid using cool-toned lights in them). Fun table lamps like lava or rock lamps can work too but keep them a few feet away from where your child sleeps. Nursery lights can help them find their comfort items and soothe themselves back to sleep more easily.

Managing lighting for specific situations can greatly support your baby's visual and overall development. Vision is one of the least developed senses in newborns, and providing consistent visual stimulation helps their retina and optic nerves mature. So, besides aiding in sleep, controlling lighting also plays a role in fostering your baby's vision development.

### The Importance of Room Temperature

Keep in mind that the temperature in your baby's room should range from 68 to 72°F. This is crucial since excessive heat raises the risk of Sudden Infant Death Syndrome (SIDS), and you should always encourage a secure sleeping environment. Due to their tiny size and ongoing growth, babies are especially sensitive to fluctuations in room temperature. But at 11 weeks, a baby's body begins to regulate its temperature at night, much like an adult's. Babies reach a minimum core body temperature of 97.5°F about four hours before bedtime.

If your baby's room lacks a thermostat, you can use an indoor thermometer to keep an eye on the temperature. However, if your baby is dressed appropriately for the weather, it is not necessary to continuously check the temperature or to keep the heating or cooling on all night.

Both toddlers and babies feel at ease at the same ambient temperature as adults do. You should dress them the same way you dress yourself—not too cold or too hot. And sometimes, they need more layers.

## Choosing the Right Crib and Bedding

Babies possess inherently sensitive skin, making them susceptible to issues like rashes and dermatitis. When these arise, it can hinder your baby's sleep despite your efforts to comfort them. Identifying the causes might require professional guidance. To prevent reaching that point, it's crucial to select appropriate bedding for your baby. Regarding the crib, as previously discussed, aside from ensuring its strength and safety, there are additional factors that need consideration.

When purchasing a crib, the foremost priority is to ensure its adherence to current safety regulations. While new cribs generally conform to these standards, if you're considering a used crib or receiving one as a gift, it's essential to meticulously examine it for compliance with the latest requirements and confirm that the manufacturer hasn't issued a recall. In acquiring a crib, it's crucial to heed the safety guidelines established by Pediatrics West, P.C. (2019):

- Any decorative cutouts on footboards and headboards are not recommended since the baby's head or limbs could become stuck there.

- The distance between crib bars should not be greater than 2 3/8 inches.

- Utilize a lead test kit to look for lead paint on antique beds.

- At least 26 inches should separate the top of the rail from the top of the bed, and as your child grows taller, you should be able to lower or adjust it.

- The top of the end panel should not be exceeded by the height of the corner post by more than 1/16 inch (1 1/2 mm). This is to prevent a baby from being strangled by their clothing catching on corner posts.

- Cribs with broken parts or missing screws should not be used.

The Centers for Disease Control and Prevention (CDC) (2019) claimed that roughly 3,500 sleep-related baby deaths occur in the United States each year, including deaths from SIDS, unintentional asphyxia, and undetermined reasons. Hence, choosing the right crib is crucial since it not only helps your baby get a good night's sleep but also ensures safety.

It's best to keep things simple when it comes to choosing bedding. A snug sheet should be used to cover mattresses. Use a flannel-backed, waterproof mattress protector or cover under the sheet, because a flannel backing is cozier and cooler than those made of rubber and plastic. Do not put blankets, padding, or pillows other than the cover between the fitted sheets and the mattress per se.

Crib bedding defines the tone and design of a nursery, and yes, it's true, but you don't want to choose anything that is beyond safety standards. The first thing you should always keep in mind is the convenience, safety, and coziness of the crib and bedding given to your little ones.

Also, don't forget to consider the room where your baby sleeps. While some parents opt to share their bed with their babies, the American Academy of Pediatrics (2022) doesn't recommend it in the first few weeks. This is because it increases the risk of SIDS, strangulation, or any other incident.

# Chapter 3:
# Establishing Healthy Sleep Habits

Establishing sleep habits for babies is quite challenging and tedious, especially for new moms. You get up every 1–2 hours a night because your baby gets fussier, which you can't understand. The worst part is that this routine may last up to two years—but fret not! Remember that nothing can replace the joy your baby brings into your life. They won't be that young forever; one day, you'll realize how time flies so fast! So, enjoy the moments of struggle during the newborn and infancy phases. But it's also good to plan things out when it comes to healthy sleep habits for you and your baby.

## The Role of Consistent Routines

Some parents let their babies do their thing in the crib or playpen until they are sleepy and fall asleep by themselves. Well, this is true only for babies who don't seem fussier. Sometimes, they make loud cries that parents can't stand, so they take them out of the crib and rock them to sleep. This is what some new parents do every time. They are just introducing a habitual ideology for babies: Every time they cry out loudly, they expect their parents to come to them and attend to their needs.

*Consistency is the key,* as they say. A bedtime routine comes with the qualities of early child stimulation and nurturing care, which are vital for positive results. Besides promoting better sleep, bedtime routines can help with literacy, language development, child behavioral and emotional control, family functioning, and parent-child connection, among others (Mindell & Williamson, 2018).

Sleep is a significant part of wellness that has an impact on many areas of early childhood development. One can get benefits from adhering to consistent bedtime routines, which include earlier bedtimes, shorter sleep latency, longer sleep durations, fewer night awakenings, and better *caregiver-reported sleep quality* (Allen et al., 2016).

While rocking or feeding your baby to sleep might seem like common bedtime routines, according to the study by Mindell & Williamson (2018), they may contribute to unhealthy sleep associations, especially in the presence of caregivers or parents, which may lead to sleep difficulties. The research highlights that the most problematic sleep patterns were associated with late bedtimes and a parent's presence while the child was falling asleep (Mindell et al., 2009). Moreover, parental presence was linked to increased night awakenings, while late bedtimes correlated with reduced overall sleep duration and prolonged sleep onset delays.

On another note, nutrition for babies can be attained with the help of consistent sleep routines. Activities including bottle or breastfeeding can improve a child's sleep, cognitive development, parent-child relationship, and overall health (Mindell & Williamson, 2018). While it was stated that parent presence negatively impacts babies' sleep, snuggling, cuddling, and rocking them *before sleep* may contribute to parent-child connection, child sleep, and emotional-behavioral control. Besides nutrition-related benefits, *communication, hygiene,* and *physical contact with parents* are greatly benefited by having a consistent sleep routine, as it promotes language development from reading bedtime stories, regular teeth brushing, and parent-child attachment, respectively.

## Developing a Bedtime Ritual

A regular bedtime routine can improve your child's sleep and reduce the number of late-night awakenings, which is good news for moms who are in dire need of a good night's sleep. To develop a bedtime ritual for your baby, the Cleveland Clinic (2023) shared six steps that you may follow:

1. Feed your baby 15 minutes before bedtime. Dr. Szugye, a Medical Director at Breastfeeding Medicine Clinic & Center, recommends feeding your baby at least 15 minutes before putting them in the crib, so they'll become drowsy and eventually fall asleep. Of course, after feeding, you don't directly put them in bed, as it may trigger any reflux. Keep them upright afterward.

2. Give them a soothing, warm bath an hour before bedtime. This is linked to a baby's body temperature as it stimulates blood circulation in their feet, arms, and extremities. Your baby's internal core cools as a result of this thermoregulatory response, a pattern connected to sleep.

3. Read a story aloud. Avoid overstimulating your baby before bedtime, limit screen time, and establish a relaxing bedtime ritual that includes activities like singing a song, reading a book, and possibly nursing—activities that will quiet and relax them.

4. Avoid screen time of all kinds. Screen time can stimulate your baby for an hour. This is because blue light from tablets, computers, phones, and televisions may inhibit melatonin production and postpone tiredness. So, stay away from these if you want your baby to sleep.

5. Establish a consistent bedtime for your baby. Do all these steps at the same time every day. Consistency is the key, and when this is established, you'll never have to worry again.

6. Also, the last thing you want to do is ensure your child is put to bed when they're drowsy but not yet asleep. This helps them learn how to fall back asleep by themselves if they ever wake up at night.

## *Nurturing Self-Soothing Skills*

You want your baby to sleep, so you sing a song and rock them to sleep while they're bottle or breastfeeding. Your baby's eyes are starting to droop, and you put them to bed because they're ready to sleep. And you wonder how long you'll have to do the same routine, or if it's infinite. It'll be endless if you do not change the way you put your baby to sleep.

Crider (2019) shared tips, medically reviewed by experts, to teach your baby to self-soothe, so you won't have to stay awake every time.

- **Know the timing**. At 3–4 months of age, many parents begin to see their baby engaging in self-soothing signs. By the time they're six months old, the majority of babies can go beyond eight hours without night feeding. It's the perfect time to teach infants to soothe themselves to sleep or go back to sleep if they wake up. Also, around this time, it's ideal to encourage self-soothing before separation anxiety becomes severe, which happens between eight and nine months. If your child already has anxiety about being separated, they may find it challenging to learn how to fall asleep on their own.

- **Keep a bedtime routine**. If you have a baby bedtime routine, keep it consistent because it helps the baby's body be aware that it's time to sleep and relax. And the next time you'll know, your baby will sleep independently at the same time.

- **Offer a soothing, safe object**. A pacifier will do for newborns for the time being. When they get older, a toy may be a replacement for it. Don't give any to newborns—including pillows and blankets—to prevent SIDS.

- **Make use of the crib**. A common practice is for babies to fall asleep in their parent's arms, which may seem comforting but can lead to undesirable sleep habits. Babies might associate sleep with being held in their parents' arms. To establish a healthier sleep routine, it's advisable to place them in the crib when they're drowsy. This way, they associate their sleeping space with the crib, making them feel at ease in their bed. If they wake up during the night, they'll likely be able to return to sleep more easily as they recognize their crib as their comfort zone.

- **Comfort the baby in their crib**. The instinct to pick up your cranky baby from the crib at night is understandable, but it's not recommended. Instead, soothe them by patting, talking, or softly singing while they remain in the crib. This practice helps both you and your baby establish a healthy sleep routine. Allowing them to learn to fall back asleep on their own is essential. It prevents the habit of needing to be carried to sleep every night for an extended period, up to a year or more.

The concept here is to be mindful of how you put your baby to sleep. Avoid allowing them to fall asleep in your arms, as this can create a habit of relying on your arms for sleep. If you've already been following this pattern, you might notice that when you place them in the crib, they start crying. This indicates that they associate sleep with being in your arms, which can become a challenging situation if you're planning to continue this for a significant portion of your parenting journey.

# Chapter 4:
# Feeding and Sleep

Breastfed infants typically require feedings every 2–3 hours, while those who are bottle-fed tend to have longer intervals of around 3–4 hours between feedings. Interestingly, even during their sleep, mothers often wake their babies up after 2–3 hours to ensure they receive their required feeding (in cases where the babies sleep longer than anticipated). Delving deeper into this practice raises the question of whether such frequent wakeups for feeding could potentially have a detrimental impact on the baby's sleep patterns. Understanding the potential effects of these feeding routines on infant sleep is an important consideration for parents seeking to strike a balance between providing necessary nourishment and ensuring their babies get adequate rest.

## Milk Feeding and Its Impact on Baby's Sleep

Getting enough sleep and food is crucial for your baby's health; they are both important for overall development. But a poorly fed baby means poor sleep habits. Food and sleep should go hand in hand because they are intertwined. If the baby keeps waking up, something might be wrong with their tummy—they may be hungry, and the recent feeding wasn't enough to make them feel better.

In the study by Brown & Harries (2015), 715 moms with children between the ages of 6 and 12 months reported regular nighttime awakenings and feedings, regardless of if it was breastmilk or any solid meals. And 78.6% continued to awaken at least once a night, with 61.4% consuming one or more night feeds. The results showed that parents who fed their babies more during the day had a lower likelihood of feeding needs at night but not of waking. This means that feeding them didn't have a significant impact on babies' sleep; they would still be awake as usual at night.

The prior study supported the research of Abdul Jafar et al. (2021), where all babies aged from 6 to 24 months still experienced night awakenings. However, fully breastfed babies had fewer instances. "Fully breastfed newborns get longer nights as well as total sleep durations than formula-fed infants."

Doctors often tell moms that newborns must only take one ounce of milk every two hours, but many parents give more than the recommended intake whenever their babies aren't at ease. According to Jain (2022), the Clinical Associate Professor of General Pediatrics and Adolescent Medicine at the University of Wisconsin School of Medicine and Public Health, babies eat every 2–3 hours, amounting to more than 12 times in 24 hours. For the first two days, newborns consume half an ounce of formula, but parents should gradually increase it in the succeeding days to 2–3 ounces every feeding time. At two months of age, they should be fed 4–5 ounces every 3–4 hours, 4–6 ounces at four months, and 6–8 ounces 4–5 times a day at six months, said the Primary Care Pediatrics at Nemours Children's Health (n.d.). If they get the right amount of intake, they won't keep bothering you every time.

However, if they're asleep at the time they should be fed, you may bottle or breastfeed them while they're sleeping so they won't need to wake up and cry out, which is a possible sign of hunger. You may also be able to sleep more than expected when they're fed well. As for breastfed babies, the recommended intake depends on their body weight, so you can give them the right amount. Always consult with your doctor about the right amount of breast milk you need to give your baby. But normally, you will convert your baby's weight (in pounds) to ounces, multiply it by 2.5, and then divide it by 8. The result is the number of ounces to be taken per bottle of breastmilk (Kotlen, 2022).

For example, if your baby's weight is 8.25 pounds, then multiply it by 2.5 (ounces). Experts recommend this amount of breast milk daily per pound of the baby's body weight up to 10 pounds, as cited in Kotlen (2022). After multiplying the body weight in pounds by 2.5, you'll get 20.6. This means your baby should be taking 20.6 ounces of breast milk in 24 hours. Since newborns need to be fed every 2–3 hours, you divide the total amount of ounces by the number of times they eat in a day. If your baby needs feeding about 8 times, then divide 20.6 by 8, and you'll get 2.6 ounces per feeding.

Ensuring your baby is well fed is just as crucial as meeting their sleep requirements. If their sleep is consistently interrupted, and they wake up frequently, especially for short periods, it could indicate hunger. Providing them with the appropriate amount of milk plays a role in achieving the necessary amount of sleep your newborn requires each day.

## Strategies for Night Feedings Without Disrupting Sleep

Now you have fed your baby the recommended milk intake. You wonder why they still wake up several times in 24 hours. You've changed their diapers and fed them again, and nothing has changed. Have you ever thought about digestive issues? This is not uncommon among babies.

### Burping

When you are done feeding your baby, make sure that you help them burp afterward. If you don't do this, the tendency is that they'll spit the milk out, which may lead to choking, especially when you accidentally fall asleep while breastfeeding (or if you ever share a bed). Your baby may swallow air while feeding, so helping them burp may take out the uncomfortable feeling, preventing acid reflux. Berry (2019) shared some effective methods on how to burp your baby, either awake or asleep.

- **Method 1**: Your baby should be positioned upright, and their head should lean against your upper chest but atop the shoulder. Place one hand beneath their buttocks as support. Pat the baby's shoulder blades gently or rub their back in a circular motion with your palm.

- **Method 2**: You may lift your baby and place them on your chest. Let them stay in a curled-up position while asleep so they won't be disturbed. With this, you have to stay awake and wait for your baby to burp. If they don't awaken, you may put them back in the crib.

- **Method 3**: The hip technique is effective for mothers who like to breastfeed their babies while in bed. You don't have to sit up, and babies are not completely in the upright position, which is a good method for burping. All you need to do is gently place your baby's tummy over the belly or hip, ensuring that the baby's head is still elevated. Pat their backs gently or in a circular motion and wait for that burping sound.

- **Method 4**: Another technique is called arm holding for *smaller babies*. Place your elbow in their crook to support their head. They might hang onto your arm with one or both of their legs. You can gently pat their back until they burp while in this posture, which applies pressure to their abdomen. This pose can be performed either sitting or standing.

- **Method 5**: Your baby should be supported on your lap with one hand under the chin  supporting their chest. Use the other hand to rub or pat the back. Gently pat your baby's back repeatedly. Make sure your baby's facing down on your lap while giving the back a light pat or stroke.

By using either one or a combination of the methods, you may help your baby release the air, preventing possible choking or any stomach discomforts after feeding.

### Dream Feeding

Willes (2017) mentioned dream feeding for babies who are younger than 16 weeks old, an instance where you feed your baby while they're asleep or half-awake. To do this, feed your baby between 9 p.m. and 10:30 p.m., while their eyes are closed. Do this every 2–3 hours because babies of this age need to be fed several times in 24 hours. If ever your baby wakes up while you attempt to dream feed them, it's okay; if it occurs every time, you may need to stop. However, if your baby stays asleep while dream feeding, you may continue to do so for the succeeding hours. It appears to work, according to some parents who tried it. As the weeks pass, their babies begin to snooze for longer, more uninterrupted stretches (Dewar, 2022). This can be supported by the study of Quante et al. (2022): Babies at six months old receiving focused bedtime meals starting at one month of age tended to slumber for longer lengths compared to those who didn't receive bedtime meals. The result showed a significant difference. Dream feeding is a good strategy to feed your sleeping baby.

In dream feeding, you must have the right timing. Remember the stages of a baby's sleep? You will only dream feed your baby once they're in active sleep, or REM. You'll know that they're in this stage when their arms and legs are moving, and their eyes lids are twitching. This way, they won't easily wake up.

If you want to try this, do not forget to use any method of burping afterward so that the baby won't be disrupted later because of the possible acid reflux.

### Feeding or Skipping

Newborns need to be fed every several hours during the 24-hour period, and it's evidence-based. However, children six months and older and those who are at least 13–14 pounds rarely need night feeds. Just because they're used to overnight feeding doesn't mean they have to be fed at this age (Willes, 2017). You have to *understand* their age and their mood whenever you feed them while they are asleep. If they're irritable once you feed them at night, you'd better skip feeding them while they're sleeping. It won't hurt them if they're not fed at night, as long as they're at the right age and have the right weight.

As newborns get older, constant feeding becomes less typical. Researchers believe that healthy, normal-weight babies don't need to be fed at night by six months old, at least not in terms of nutrition (Ruggeri, 2022). Look at the baby to determine what is best for them, whether it is a tight schedule built on 7:7 sleep or something else. It's better to understand them first if they're fine with night feeds.

Breastfed babies wake up when they're hungry every 2–3 hours because they easily digest milk. However, formula-fed babies may go around 3–4 hours since formula takes a little longer to digest.

Before they get to the part where they make loud cries, you may want to dream feed your baby so that their sleep won't be interrupted. Make sure they're asleep while you do it, in active sleep. Once you're done feeding, you may use a burping strategy, so they won't get sick as they doze off.

In case they're awake while you feed them at night, be gentle. Continue having that sleep-conducive environment: a dimmed room with white noise. Add to that your gentle pat while singing them a lullaby or softly talking with them. This may calm them and help them fall back to sleep.

# Solid Foods and Their Effect on Sleep Patterns

You might have heard that babies can start consuming solid food around the age of six months. Nevertheless, this doesn't imply that you should introduce any food your baby seems to enjoy. Occasionally, babies who try solid foods or even drinks, like shakes or juice, for the first time become quite fond of them and seek more. While it's tempting to give in to their requests, it's not advisable, as certain foods can potentially disrupt their digestive system and impact their wellbeing for days. Moreover, this might lead to frequent visits to your pediatrician for medications and follow-ups.

The initial meals should be finely mashed or smooth, depending on their preferences. In the upcoming weeks and months, your baby can progress to roughly mashed or minced foods and eventually chopped foods. The key is to ensure everything has a soft texture. Babies need exposure to various food textures (Raising Children Network, 2023), which helps them learn how to chew effectively. This also plays a role in preventing feeding difficulties as your baby grows. By the time they reach 12 months old, they should be consuming similar foods as adults, although you might need to chop or mince the foods to maintain their softness.

The food you introduce to your baby can also impact their sleep, so you need to be cautious with your food choices. While some babies may tolerate various food textures, others can be sensitive. Sensitivity in babies might not be immediately apparent, and you'll only notice it if they react negatively to certain foods. The best way to discern this is by introducing new foods in small portions. If there's a positive response, you can proceed with feeding. Otherwise, it's better to discontinue. How can you determine if your baby is having an allergic reaction to the food you're giving them?

Shaw (2023) of WebMD said that parents should always watch for symptoms of allergic reactions when introducing solid food to babies, which are as follows:

- wheezing or coughing

- diarrhea and/or spitting out

- flushed skin

- welts/hives

- loses sense of consciousness

- difficulty breathing

If an allergy is present, it can significantly affect your baby's health, leading to irritability both during the day and at night. You certainly don't want to experience the same sluggishness, especially when you need to be awake all night attending to your baby's discomfort. While frustration and exhaustion might arise, ultimately, caregivers need to take responsibility for the food they provide to their little ones.

If you have a family history of allergies, always see your doctor, and talk about it before introducing them to solid foods. Most allergenic foods are shellfish, cow's milk, peanuts, wheat, eggs, and more.

If you are breastfeeding, continue it up to 12 months of age because it is still the main source of nutrients. To avoid sleep issues with your baby, avoid the following foods and drinks (Raising Children Network, 2023):

- **Honey**: Don't introduce them to honey until they're at least 12 months of age because it may lead to infant botulism—a potentially fatal condition or toxins produced by the bacteria *Clostridium botulinum*. These microorganisms can contaminate several foods, including honey.

- **Runny or raw eggs**: Eggs that are runny or raw should not be given to infants under 12 months due to the dangers of the bacteria residing in them.

- **Low-fat milk**: Not until they're 12 months old because they need to gain weight.

- **Hard, solid foods**: Nuts, candies, grapes, and the like are choking hazards.

- **Pasteurized cow's milk**: Whether full-fat or skimmed milk, avoid it as the *primary* milk supply. Formulas are okay since they're pasteurized according to the baby's needs.

- **Dairy substitutes**: Not until the age of two, avoid dairy substitutes including sheep, goat, rice, soy, oat, coconut, and almond milk unless your doctor has specifically advised it.

- **Unpasteurized milk**: Unpasteurized milk is raw milk in which bacteria may still be present. Choose milk that's specifically processed for babies.

- **Fruit juices**: They should be kept to a minimum (whole fruits are preferable because they provide fiber and aid in the development of feeding and chewing skills in infants).

- **Sugary or sweetened drinks, tea, and coffee**: You know this isn't suggested at any age.

When giving solid food to babies, it is important to take developmental readiness, choking concerns, and other health problems into account. To promote a secure, healthy, and successful transition to solid foods, parents should speak with their pediatrician and follow the advice given.

Also, it is significant to note that a variety of elements, such as teething, developmental milestones, and adjustments in feeding habits, can influence a baby's sleep. While introducing solid food may not necessarily improve sleep, it is important to follow recommended guidelines, give correct solid foods when the baby is developmentally ready, and be mindful of any changes in sleep patterns.

# Chapter 5:
# Navigating Nap Times

No amount of words can express the joy parents feel when they see their little ones sleeping so soundly. And this holds even more true when they fall asleep just when you have so much to do!

When their eyes are drooping, you sense some "me" time—where you can relax for a bit or tend to something important while they're asleep. The challenge arises when your baby finds it difficult to nod off. You could spend half a day trying to help them snooze. This is a demanding task for mothers, but the knowledge of how to put your precious ones to sleep—for your physical and emotional wellbeing—is truly something to celebrate!

## *Age-Appropriate Nap Schedules*

Newborns take time to establish a sleep pattern because their circadian rhythms need time to develop. They'll sleep for about 16 hours each day for the first month. Typically, this takes the form of 3–4 nap cycles between feedings. After being awake for 1–2 hours, they'll go back to sleep. Nap times usually become more predictable as they age (Mayo Clinic Staff, 2022).

- **From four months up to one year old**. Following the initial newborn phase, it's likely that your infant will take two naps daily, usually in the morning and early afternoon. Some babies might need an extra nap later in the afternoon. You might consider scheduling your baby's naps for 9 a.m. and 1 p.m. Allow your baby to nap for their preferred duration, unless nighttime sleep proves challenging. If your baby takes a third nap in the late afternoon, it's advisable to phase it out around the nine-month mark. This adjustment can help prepare your baby for an earlier bedtime routine.

- **For ages one year and older**. As your baby reaches nine months to one year old, a morning nap will no longer be necessary. While navigating this transition, think about advancing your baby's nap time and bedtime by around 30 minutes to ease the adjustment. Typically, children continue to take an afternoon nap lasting 1–2 hours until around the age of three. After this stage, the nap duration usually shortens.

Nap schedules vary significantly among different infants. However, when considering nap durations, babies generally fall into two primary categories: the *extended nappers*, who enjoy napping for 2–3 hours, and the *brief nappers*, who have shorter nap durations—sometimes as brief as 30 minutes—but may experience more frequent periods of rest during the day. Further information on nap schedules for babies is provided by O'Connor (2022):

- At three months old, you can expect three to four naps daily, each lasting between 30 minutes and 2 hours.

- Moving on to four months old, anticipate two or three naps daily, with each nap spanning one to two hours.

- By the time your baby reaches five months old, continue with two to three naps daily, each ranging from one to two hours.

- As your baby hits the six-month mark, maintain a routine of two to three naps daily, each extending from one to two hours.

- For babies aged 7 to 12 months, settle into a pattern of two naps daily—one in the morning and another in the afternoon—each lasting around one to two hours.

In addition, make sure to follow appropriate wake intervals for your baby between naps, based on their age in months:

- In the first month, maintain a 45-minute gap between naps.

- Ages 1–2 months: Allow 45 to 60 minutes between naps.

- Ages 2–4 months: Aim for a wake time of 1.5–3 hours.

- Ages 5–8 months: Opt for a wake time of 2.5–3 hours.

- Ages 9–12 months: Extend the wake intervals to 2.5–4 hours.

While these schedules for baby naps can offer guidance, it's important to note that there are no strict, fixed rules regarding the duration of a baby's naps.

As long as your baby is meeting the recommended daily sleep hours, there's no need to be concerned about the length of their naps. However, excessively long naps in the late afternoon might potentially disrupt nighttime sleep for older babies, requiring adjustments to their nap routine to ensure they're prepared for bedtime.

## Transitioning From Multiple Naps to Fewer Naps

The shift from having multiple naps to fewer naps is a significant developmental step for babies, signifying a crucial change in their sleep cycles. As infants mature and their sleep requirements transform, the progression from frequent short naps to a more consolidated nap schedule becomes pivotal in establishing healthy sleep routines. Although this transition is a natural evolution, it demands careful attention and adjustments to ensure a smooth and seamless adaptation process.

Willes (2017) provided insights into guiding mothers through the process of transitioning their infants from having several naps to reducing the number of naps.

### The 3-2 Transition

Willes (2017) stated that navigating the transition from three naps to two can be a challenging process. Your child may be ready to move to two naps when:

- They are no longer falling asleep for all three naps (due to reduced tiredness for the third nap).

- While they manage to fall asleep for all three naps, they struggle to fall asleep at bedtime, wake up during the night, or wake up too early in the morning without being able to go back to sleep.

- They can fall asleep three times a day, but the third nap extends beyond 4 p.m.

When you decide it's time to transition to two naps, adjust your child's nap schedule to 9 a.m. and 1:30 p.m., while also considering an earlier bedtime if necessary. Typically, this transition lasts around 7–10 days, so it's crucial to remain consistent and avoid switching back and forth between three and two naps.

### The 2-1 Transition

When the time comes to transition your toddler to a single nap per day, it's important to note that it will take approximately 30 days for them to consolidate all their daytime sleep into this one nap.

Throughout this month-long period, refrain from introducing a second nap solely based on the length of your child's initial nap, even if it's just 45 minutes. Instead, maintain wakefulness until bedtime, considering an earlier bedtime by 30 minutes, but avoid switching back and forth between one and two naps.

Managing nap schedule adjustments at this stage is relatively uncomplicated. You have the option to make an abrupt change by having your child stay awake until around 11 a.m., allowing them to nod off, and then keeping them awake until their regular bedtime. Alternatively, you can make gradual changes by shifting their first nap to 15 minutes later every 2–3 days. Additionally, continue to have them rest in their crib with lights off and white noise on for about 30 minutes around 2 p.m. each day, even if they don't sleep but simply *rest*. Once the initial nap is set for 11 a.m., discontinue the afternoon nap and progressively adjust the timing of the 11 a.m. nap until it begins at a suitable time for your child—usually between 12 and 1 p.m. for most children.

Here's another set of suggestions aimed at assisting your baby's transition to a single daily nap, as outlined by O'Connor (2023) in her article *How to Transition from Two Naps to One*.

- Gradually extend the period of time your baby stays awake in the morning. Allow them to remain awake for a minimum of four to five hours before their afternoon nap.

- Adjust the timing of lunch and dinner if they seem excessively drowsy. This will enable you to initiate your afternoon nap earlier and establish a bedtime that's also earlier.

- Incorporate a peaceful interval during their usual morning nap time. If they appear irritable or fatigued during their typical morning nap, replace it with a mid-morning quiet interlude involving books and comforting moments.

- Make sure your baby's afternoon nap lasts around 1 to 2.5 hours. If your baby has outgrown morning naps, they might need a shorter afternoon nap. If their nap is shorter than two hours, make sure they're sleeping well at night and talk to your doctor if you're worried. You could explore sleep training for naps or try a calming routine before nap time.

- If you notice your child getting crankier as the evening comes, try moving their bedtime earlier. Shifting their sleep schedule to an earlier time might help as they adapt to their new single-nap routine.

Therefore, transitioning a baby from multiple naps to fewer naps is an important and natural phase in their development. As babies grow and their sleep patterns change, this shift plays a vital role in setting up healthy sleep habits.

## Encouraging Longer and More Restful Naps

Every parent wants their baby to be good at taking naps. A study by Tham et al. (2017) showed that there is a favorable connection between sleep, language, memory, cognitive development, and executive function in typically developing infants and young children. Hence, taking naps has benefits for your baby, but establishing a successful nap routine can be challenging.

As mentioned earlier, babies vary; not all can nap when parents desire them to. Some remain active both during the day and throughout the night. Others sleep during the day but become nocturnal, leading parents to experience frustration and struggle. Parents need to understand the distinction between short and long naps. According to LoRe (2023), short naps occur when babies sleep for 45 minutes or less—a single sleep cycle. Conversely, longer naps lasting 1.5 to 3 hours happen when babies progress through multiple sleep cycles.

If your infant is having difficulty with extended nap times, it's essential to examine potential factors that might be causing their naps to be brief. If they have already received sufficient rest, even if it's earlier than you prefer, there might not be many options. However, if your baby is waking up due to other factors that hinder their sleep duration, there are strategies you can employ to promote longer naps.

The solution might be as straightforward as establishing a consistent nap routine early on and sticking to it. Utilizing dim lights and a quiet story can assist children in easing into nap time.

Place infants into their cribs when they're feeling drowsy but not yet asleep. This helps them develop the ability to fall asleep independently, a skill that becomes even more vital as they grow older.

For preschoolers and toddlers, set regular nap times that are spaced reasonably apart from their bedtime. Adhering to a fixed nap schedule can present a challenge. While many still enjoy their naps, some resist sleep to avoid missing out on anything. If your child discontinues daytime naps, consider establishing an earlier bedtime. Normally, your child sleeps early and wakes up early too.

Here's another suggestion provided by Zwarensteyn (2020) from her article *How to Get Your Baby to Nap Longer—Learn Useful Tips And Tricks*:

- **Avoid noises**. Loud noises like barking puppies, sirens, or ringing phones can disturb a baby's sleep. Control what you can by silencing your phone, using a baby monitor, and maintaining a comfortable room temperature for uninterrupted sleep.

- **Establish sleep routines**. Infants experience brief sleep cycles, typically lasting around 50–60 minutes, during which they spend a greater portion of their time in light sleep. Frequently, they awaken while transitioning between these cycles. Monitor their waking moments to gauge the duration of each cycle.

- **No screen time**. Resist the urge to let them watch screens before naps, as their active minds might stay awake despite turning off the device. Also, you might want to avoid this, as babies tend to become captivated by the lights emitted from electronic devices.

- **Give your infant a snack before bedtime**. Babies and little kids grow quickly, and sometimes they seem to be hungry all the time. Have you ever wondered where all that food goes? If your child is feeling hungry, they might struggle to fall asleep. And even if they do fall asleep, a growling tummy or hunger pang could wake them up too soon. To help them sleep better, try giving them a small snack before their nap time. This gives their tummies time to digest the food before they lay down for a nap.

- **Pay attention to your baby's signals**. Watch both the clock and how your baby acts. If your baby seems tired—like yawning, rubbing their eyes, or looking sleepy—it's time for a nap. Put them in their special sleep spot, like their crib, without toys or blankets, as soon as you can. With time, you'll get to know your baby's schedule and can plan what you do based on that.

- **Start using a white noise machine**. If your home is really noisy (maybe your baby's nap time overlaps with the next-door high school band practicing in the garage), you'll want something to block out the noise. A white noise machine could help. It also makes a soothing whooshing sound, like what babies hear in the womb.

Encouraging healthy nap routines is crucial for a baby's wellbeing and growth. Create a comfy sleep environment, heed their cues, and consider techniques like white noise or light snacks. These practices lead to peaceful naps and happier, more alert babies, setting the stage for positive sleep habits and overall development.

# Chapter 6:
# Sleep Training Methods

Taking care of your little ones and making sure they sleep well can be tough. It's confusing to know what to do first and next. When your baby keeps waking up and crying, so do you, especially if you're a new mom. But crying along with your baby doesn't help. The good news is that some ways and tips can help your baby sleep better. These methods are based on science and advice from sleep experts and are tailored to your needs.

## Introduction to Well-Known Sleep Training Techniques

Parents should know about sleep training methods for their babies because it helps them establish good sleep routines, which is important for their growth.

Knowing these methods gives you some ways to handle common sleep issues like waking up often or having an irregular sleep schedule. By learning different approaches, you can choose what works best for your family and your baby. It also makes your home more peaceful and improves sleep for both you and your baby.

### The Ferber Method

According to Taylor (2023), The Ferber method, also called *graduated extinction*, was created by Dr. Richard Ferber, an expert in pediatric sleep. With this technique, parents let their children learn to fall asleep on their own, comforting them at intervals. It helps babies learn self-soothing and sleep independently, even when they wake up at night. Some parents who use *cry-it-out* (CIO) for sleep training choose not to return to their baby's room, even if the baby cries for a while. The Ferber method is a gentler option, where you check on your baby at certain times while they cry.

During these checks, you visit your baby at gradually increasing intervals until they fall asleep. The time between checks also gets longer on later nights, which Ferber calls the *progressive waiting approach*. You can talk soothingly or give a gentle pat. But you shouldn't pick your baby up or feed them, and your visits should only last a minute or two.

Dr. Richard Ferber, after whom the Ferber method is named, is a medical professional who serves as the Director at The Center for Pediatric Sleep Disorders, situated at Children's Hospital Boston. With over three decades of experience, he has devoted his research to the examination of sleep and sleep-related concerns in children (Encyclopedia, n.d.).

### The Weissbluth Method

Dr. Marc Weissbluth, known for his book *Healthy Sleep Habits, Happy Child,* believes a child's sleep patterns reveal their overall wellbeing. He suggests parents can use routines to improve sleep habits. Although sometimes mixed up with the Ferber method, the Weissbluth approach to sleep training is quite different. Learning about the Weissbluth method can help you decide if it's the right fit for you (Education.com, 2012).

Some parents confuse the Weissbluth method with Ferber because both involve letting their child cry a bit to learn self-soothing. But there's a difference: the Ferber method has parents comforting at intervals, while Weissbluth has no comforting at all to stop nighttime waking and crying. With Weissbluth, parents should put their children to bed early and only enter the room for emergencies. He also suggests longer sleep at night, even if daytime naps are shorter or fewer.

Weissbluth says his method works faster than Ferberizing because babies realize sooner that their cries won't get a response. His approach takes around 3–4 days, while Ferber's can take up to two weeks. This method also involves paying attention to when your baby seems tired and putting her to sleep right away, which is helpful for all parents. However, some parents find it sad to hear their baby cry all night. Ignoring their cries completely might make them feel helpless, and it doesn't consider other reasons like being sick, changes in routine, hunger, or fear.

### The Murkoff Method

Heidi Murkoff wrote the popular pregnancy guide series *What to Expect When You're Expecting*. She also created *WhatToExpect.com* and started the *What to Expect Project.*

Heidi Murkoff says that when babies are around four months old, or weighing about 11 lbs., they begin to sleep longer without night feedings. Sleep training can begin at this age and includes things like graduated extinction, making sleep patterns better, and scheduled awakenings (Marcin, 2023).

Parents can start sleep training methods like graduated extinction, scheduled awakening, and reinforcing sleep routines after the baby turns four months. At six months, Murkoff suggests a *cold turkey* approach to CIO.

### The Baby Whisperer Method

Tracy Hogg, a British nurse and successful author, died when she was 44. Her time working in different hospitals, including St. Catherine's Hospital for the Mentally Handicapped, shaped her knowledge of taking care of children. On the other hand, Melinda Blau, known for her popular books like the *Secrets of Baby Whisperer* series, partnered with Hogg to create *the Hogg and Blau Method*, also called the Baby Whisperers. Their method offers helpful ideas for teaching babies to sleep well.

Tracy Hogg, known as the "baby whisperer," and Melinda Blau suggest that babies can sleep through the night once they weigh around 10 pounds. They recommend feeding them more in the evenings and doing a dream feed. The authors talk about three stages of crying, or *crescendos,* before sleep. Parents usually give in during the second peak of crying. Their approach lets parents comfort their baby but advises leaving once the baby starts calming down (Marcin, 2023).

### The Giordano and Abidin Method

Suzy Giordano, a mother of five, is affectionately known as *the Baby Coach* for her work in Washington, DC. On the flip side, Lisa Abidin—a mother of twins—has experience as a prosecutor and law clerk. Both authors have written books on sleep training with similar concepts, giving rise to the term Giordano and Abidin method.

Suzy Giordano and Lisa Abidin believe that by the time babies are 12 weeks old, they can sleep for 12 hours straight without needing a nighttime feed. Starting at eight weeks of age, their method involves letting the baby cry for three to five minutes at night before responding. Instead of feeding at night, the authors recommend parents feed babies every three hours during the day (Marcin, 2023).

### *The Bucknam and Ezzo Method*

Authors Robert Bucknam, MD, and Gary Ezzo, in their book on *Becoming Baby-wise*, highlight the importance of teaching babies to soothe themselves, a gift with lasting advantages. They suggest that babies as young as seven to nine weeks can sleep for around eight hours at night, which increases to 11 hours by the time they're 12 weeks old. This involves letting the baby cry for 15 to 20 minutes before going to sleep. It's also essential to follow a specific daytime sleep routine, e.g., *eat*, then *wake* and *sleep*.

Generally, these methods fall under the umbrella term "cry it out." The CIO method, also called controlled crying, is a way to teach babies to sleep on their own. Research by Mindell et al. (2006) showed that using this method can help improve a baby's long-term sleep patterns and ability to handle stress. It encourages independence in babies and gives parents a chance to rest and focus when the baby is awake. It allows short-term stress for long-term benefits.

Now, if you can't stand letting your baby cry for a minute, then you may try Elizabeth Pantley's.

### *The No-Cry Sleep Solution Method*

Elizabeth Pantley wrote a book called *The No-Cry Sleep Solution*. It helps parents and caregivers make their children sleep better without using the CIO. The book gives tips for creating good sleep habits for babies and young kids. The main idea of the *No-Cry Sleep Solution* is to be kind, patient, and understanding when dealing with sleep problems. Every child is different, so the book offers different ways to gently improve sleep, reduce disruptions, and teach kids how to soothe themselves (SnoozeShade, n.d.).

She talks about things like creating a cozy sleep environment, having a regular bedtime routine, knowing when your child is tired, and helping them learn to calm down on their own. The book says it's important for parents to respond to their child's needs and to make sleep training less stressful. The method is just one way to help kids sleep better. It's good for parents who don't want to use methods where the child cries a lot.

## *Selecting the Method Aligned With Your Parenting Style*

One of the first things new parents quickly realize is that the saying *sleeping like a baby* isn't always true. While some lucky parents have babies who sleep well at night, many others face sleep challenges.

To deal with this, many parents try sleep training, a method to teach kids how to sleep independently. But there's a lot of advice out there, sometimes contradictory, about how to do sleep training. This can lead to strong opinions among parents, making it a bit tricky to navigate.

Hence, how you teach your baby to sleep better *depends on what you like and how your baby acts*. It might be helpful to learn about different methods and ask a doctor before choosing the one that's right for your family. "I suggest taking a balanced approach," advises Dr. Wendy Nash, a clinical psychiatrist at the Child Mind Institute. "Rather than responding to each night separately, it's better to observe patterns and recurring issues." Sleep disruptions can often be due to growth spurts or teething, but if they persist for more than a couple of weeks, considering sleep training would be a suitable option, as cited in Martinelli (2023).

The age at which it's best to begin sleep training can vary a lot, from three months to even more than a year old. Usually, around six months is a good time, but it's smart to talk to your doctor too. This way, you can make sure your baby is growing well and getting enough food during the day. Also, you may then apply the proper sleep training method for your baby according to your parenting style.

### Parenting Style and Sleep Training

Ultimately, your approach to sleep training hinges on your parenting style. As a parent, it's tough to see your child crying and unable to sleep. But sleep training, like coaching them to sleep better, can help (if there are no other reasons why babies can't nod off). Navigating the sleep coaching journey can be demanding, and your particular parenting approach plays a part. Now, let's look at the different parenting styles of Adair (2023) and how they might affect helping your baby sleep better.

### Attachment Parenting Approach

Attachment parenting is about being close to your child and always being there for them. This can help kids feel safe and sleep better. With this style, you might take more time to help your child learn to sleep on their own without crying. But in the end, it can make your bond with your child stronger and create a good sleeping routine.

### Authoritative Approach

Authoritative parenting is when parents balance rules with being caring. This can help a child sleep better because the parents have clear rules and routines. When it's time to teach a child to sleep well, this style can work well because the child is used to routines, which makes learning to sleep easier and more effective.

### Authoritarian Approach

Authoritarian parenting means strict rules and watching your child closely. This can help them learn rules and routines. But when it comes to sleep coaching, it can be a problem. Authoritarian parents think a child's crying is just a trick, so sleep training with crying might be hard for them. This could make sleep training take longer and be tough for both the parent and child. Or, if they use a method like controlled crying, it might make the training shorter because the parent doesn't quickly attend to the child's cries.

### Permissive Approach

Permissive parenting means letting the child do whatever they want without many rules. Of all the parenting styles mentioned, this one can make the child's sleep schedule irregular and cause sleep problems later. Regarding sleep training, permissive parenting can be hard because the parent isn't used to setting rules. The biggest problem is that there's no consistent routine in the child's life.

Before you begin sleep coaching with your child, it's crucial to understand your parenting style. Pick a method that feels good for you and your baby. Try it for a few weeks. If it doesn't work, take a break for a couple of weeks. Then, you can try again or choose a different way.

## Step-by-Step Guides to Different Training Techniques

You've already grasped the seven sleep training methods and when to apply them according to your parenting style. As parents and caregivers, you're always on the lookout for effective ways to assist your children in growing and thriving. Visualizing the steps of your chosen sleep training method might be a challenge, so exploring each method and doing detailed walkthroughs may help you begin.

### *The Ferber Method*

Although sleep training might be emotionally challenging, the actual steps of the Ferber method are simple and direct. Here's what you'll do:

- Once you've finished your bedtime routine, place your baby in the crib. Your baby should be somewhat sleepy but still awake.

- Say goodnight to your baby and exit the room.

- If your baby starts crying, wait for a specific amount of time, then return briefly to soothe her by speaking softly or gently patting her. Avoid picking her up or feeding her.

- Leave the room and repeat this process. If your baby continues to cry, return at designated intervals to offer reassurance.

The Ferber method is a gentler way of doing CIO sleep training. You check on your crying baby at set times to comfort her.

In his book, *Solve Your Child's Sleep Problems*, Ferber, as cited by Taylor (2023), suggests checking in at these times:

Day 1

- First check-in: 3 minutes

- Second check-in: 5 minutes

- Third check-in: 10 minutes

- After: 10 minutes

Day 2

- First check-in: 5 minutes

- Second check-in: 10 minutes

- Third check-in: 12 minutes

- After: 12 minutes

Day 3

- First check-in: 10 minutes

- Second check-in: 12 minutes

- Third check-in: 15 minutes

- After: 15 minutes

Day 4

- First check-in: 12 minutes

- Second check-in: 15 minutes

- Third check-in: 17 minutes

- After: 17 minutes

Day 5

- First check-in: 15 minutes

- Second check-in: 17 minutes

- Third check-in: 20 minutes

- After: 20 minutes

Day 6

- First check-in: 17 minutes

- Second check-in: 20 minutes

- Third check-in: 25 minutes

- After: 25 minutes

Day 7

- First check-in: 20 minutes

- Second check-in: 25 minutes

- Third check-in: 30 minutes

- After: 30 minutes

The Ferber method helps your baby learn to sleep on their own and soothe themselves at night. There might be some tears, like with many sleep training methods.


### The Weissbluth Method

Before using the Weissbluth method, consult your doctor, especially if your baby is under six months old and still wakes up for changing and feeding. Once you get approval, here's how to do it (Education.com, 2012):

- Put your baby in the crib when they show signs of tiredness, like rubbing their eyes or being fussy.

- Let them make noise in the crib; avoid rocking or feeding them to sleep. Stick to a routine.

- Leave the room, even if they cry. Listen nearby, but don't comfort them. They'll learn to fall asleep on their own.

- Stick to a consistent nap schedule, focusing more on nighttime sleep.

- Stay consistent. The Weissbluth method works quickly if they're ready. If you give in, try again or pick a sleep method that suits your parenting style.

The Weissbluth method is a choice for promoting healthy sleep habits in babies. It helps them learn to sleep on their own and have longer, more restful sleep. This method focuses on consistency and routine, aiming for better sleep patterns. Again, before applying, consider if your baby is ready and if it fits your parenting style. Consulting a doctor can help you decide if it's right for your baby's sleep needs.

### The Murkoff Method

Murkoff's method focuses on *reducing night feedings* to help babies sleep better, and it's recommended to start around 4 months of age or when they reach 11 pounds. While there is no detailed step-by-step guide available, the RCN (2022) discussed sleep training ideas in two separate sections for breastfed and formula-fed babies that aligned with Murkoff's.

### Gradual Transition from Nighttime Breastfeeding

Night weaning means helping your baby stop waking up for nighttime feedings. Your baby will have the first feeding when she wakes up in the morning, continue to feed during the day, and have the last feeding just before going to bed. This is how it works:

- Quick Night Feeds

If your baby's nighttime feed is brief (under five minutes), you can gradually stop it. Use your preferred sleep methods to help your baby settle. It might take a few nights to adjust.

- Extended Night Feeds

For longer nighttime feeds, gradually reduce time over 5–7 nights:

- Trim feeding time by 2–5 minutes every other night.

- Settle your baby after shorter feeds.

- If upset, pause the weaning process briefly.

*Key Things to Remember*

- If you try night weaning, remember that your child still benefits from unlimited breastfeeding during the day.

- During big changes, your child might want more comfort and food.

- If your child seeks nighttime comfort but is not feeding, your partner could help soothe them at night.

### Easing Night Feedings for Formula-Fed Babies

For babies who are given formula, you might think about slowly giving them fewer night feedings when they reach six months.

Once formula-fed babies are over six months old, they probably won't wake up at night because they're hungry. This is because formula takes longer to digest than breast milk.

- Nighttime Feedings With Less Than 60 mL of Milk

If you're thinking of stopping nighttime feeds and your baby drinks 60 mL of milk or less, you can skip the feed and use your preferred calming techniques to soothe your baby.

- Nighttime Feedings With More Than 60 mL of Milk

For babies consuming more than 60 mL of milk in their nighttime feed, you can gradually reduce the amount over 5–7 nights.

Here's how:

- Lower the milk quantity by 20–30 mL every second night. For example, if your baby usually has 180 mL, provide 150 mL for two nights, then 120 mL for the next two nights, and so forth.

- Comfort your baby with your chosen settling methods after each smaller feed.

Once the milk amount reaches 60 mL or less, you can discontinue the nighttime feed entirely.

Gradually reducing nighttime feeds can be a thoughtful process for both breastfed and formula-fed babies. Consider your baby's needs and your style. Whether it's for better sleep or adjusting to growth, these strategies can help. Remember, every baby is different, so find what works best for your family. And don't forget to consult your healthcare provider for guidance along the way.

### The Baby Whisperer Method

The *pickup, put down* sleep training method is quite simple. It comes from Tracy Hogg's *Secrets of the Baby Whisperer* book. Many parents find this sleep training method gentle because it helps babies learn to soothe themselves without leaving them alone to cry in their cribs.

Tracy created a *pickup, put down* for babies who struggle to sleep. Here's how it works: If your baby cries, you go to them and use gentle words and touches on their tummy to calm them. If they keep crying, you pick them up to comfort them, then put them back in the crib once they're calm. You can comfort them with words or touches, and if necessary, pick them up again without rocking them to sleep. Repeat this until they fall asleep. The goal is to let your baby know you're there if they need you, and they'll learn to sleep on their own over time (Geddes, 2022).

### The Giordano and Abidin Method

Suzy Giordano, also known as *The Child Coach*, along with Lisa Abidin, developed a method to help babies sleep through the night by the age of 12 weeks. This technique teaches babies the difference between daytime and nighttime, encouraging wakefulness during the day and minimal interaction at night. Here's how it's implemented:

- Keep track of when your baby eats and sleeps for the first eight weeks.

- Create a schedule based on your baby's natural patterns using this information.

- Aim for daytime feedings every four hours, with the last four-hour stretch keeping your baby awake except for a quick nap.

- Start adjusting the schedule at eight weeks. If your baby wants to eat earlier, gently distract them until closer to feeding time.

- Once the new schedule is set, gradually reduce nighttime feedings by giving less food until they're no longer needed. Stick to the schedule and soothe your baby until feeding time.

- After stopping nighttime feedings, encourage your baby to sleep in the crib for 12 hours. It's okay if they cry for short periods; soothe them and repeat until they can sleep for 12 hours straight (Gold, 2017).

The 12 Hours by 12 Weeks Method offers a structured approach to improving a baby's sleep. By adjusting schedules and promoting longer nighttime rest, parents can help establish healthy sleep patterns. Remember, patience and consistency are vital for success.

### *The Bucknam and Ezzo Method*

The Bucknam and Ezzo Method is a simple, step-by-step guide to improving your baby's sleep. Whether you're a new parent or looking to enhance your routine, the technique offers practical tips for healthier sleep habits. Here's how you do it:

- Use the eat-wake-sleep pattern. Once your baby knows day and night, teach them to fall asleep on their own when they're a bit awake. This is like the easy schedule in other sleep books and helps prevent nursing sleep problems later.

- Make sure the baby gets full feedings. Because your baby isn't falling asleep while feeding, they eat enough and sleep longer.

- Watch for signs. When your baby is tired, track wake times, and adjust nap times when needed.

- Wake the baby up to eat. Baby-wise parents don't always follow the rule of *never waking a sleeping baby*. They wake babies to feed them more during the day for better nighttime sleep and the right amount of daytime sleep (Motroni, 2019).

By following these patterns and schedules, babies can have better naps, sleep longer at night, and the whole family can have a predictable routine to follow.

### *The No-Cry Sleep Solution Method*

In Elizabeth Pantley's well-known book, the *no-cry* approach is about adapting to your baby's needs.

Remember (Netmums, 2016):

- Comfort and feed your baby until sleepy before placing them down.

- If they cry, pick them up right away.

Essential to this gentle method is a consistent bedtime routine and understanding your baby's sleep patterns. This can be achieved by:

- Keeping track of your baby's patterns to understand their sleep needs and prevent unnecessary tears.

- Creating a consistent sleep routine that matches your baby's natural body clock is especially important after 3–4 months.

- Knowing how long your baby usually sleeps at different ages and remember that waking up at night is normal before 12 months.

- Watching for signs of tiredness and starting calming routines 15 minutes before their usual bedtime.

- Making a peaceful sleep environment by maintaining a comfortable room temperature (68–72°F), using blackout blinds, and trying white noise if it helps.

- Using calming words like *sleepy time* or *shh* when putting your baby down, similar to the *pickup, put down* method.

- Learning your baby's cries to tell if they need comfort or if they're just falling asleep.

In the quest for better baby sleep, remember each child is different. Whether you use specific methods or a mix, be patient, consistent, and attentive to their needs. Understand sleep patterns, create a calming environment, and respond to cues for healthy sleep habits. This journey leads to peaceful nights and happy days for your baby and family.

# Chapter 7:
# Addressing Sleep Disruptions

Parenthood—a magical journey filled with giggles and first discoveries—introduces a curious nighttime challenge: sleep disruptions in babies. Just like a gentle breeze carries whispers through the night, these disruptions can make peaceful sleep a bit tricky for both babies and tired parents.

During those early months of life, when everything is new and fascinating, sleep disruptions often pop up like little surprises. They're like friendly shadows that tag along during the night, making sleep a bit of a puzzle for babies and their loving parents. While cuddles and lullabies create heartwarming moments, figuring out a baby's sleep can sometimes feel like solving a cozy mystery.

Getting to know these sleep disruptions is important. They're like hints that babies give you, telling you how they're feeling. By understanding these hints, you can learn to read the signs and find ways to make nights more peaceful for you and everyone else.

## Teething, Growing Spurts, and Developmental Milestones

Parenthood struggles can endure for years. As they say, once children come into the world, parents often find themselves sleep-deprived until their children reach adulthood. Adequate sleep becomes a rarity for parents. Amidst various teething issues in children, it has been revealed that symptoms can affect a significant portion of the children studied, with some studies reporting rates as high as 80–90%. The findings from this specific study indicate that 68% of children experiencing tooth eruption exhibited general systemic symptoms, such as drooling, fever, and diarrhea, while 32% of the sample showed no noticeable symptoms. With this matter, you can consider teething as one of the culprits for why your baby can't sleep no matter what you do.

### Teething

Teething starts when babies are around 4–8 months old, often starting with their bottom front teeth. It keeps going until they're about 30 to 36 months old, and that's when their last molars come in. While babies are teething, they might show signs like being fussier, drooling a lot, not wanting to eat as much, having swollen or red gums, getting a rash near their mouth, having looser stools, having a little fever, rubbing their gums, biting things more, and sometimes pulling at their ears.

It's hard to ignore baby teething, especially since it makes them irritable 24 hours a day. So, if you can't see a doctor because it's late at night or you live far from the city, you may try the following for the time being (*Teething: Tips for Soothing Sore Gums,* 2018):

- **Gently rub your baby's gums**. You can use a clean finger or a slightly wet cloth to massage their gums, which can help make them feel better.

- **Keep things cool**. A teething ring that's been chilled in the fridge (not frozen) or a cold spoon can give relief to their gums. But don't put anything sugary on them to avoid worsening of teething.

- **Think about over-the-counter options**. If your child is fussy, you can think about giving them over-the-counter pain medicines for children, like acetaminophen or ibuprofen.

Providing additional comfort can be highly beneficial if your baby becomes distressed due to teething during the night. Offer a comforting hug or gentle rocking to help your baby relax and ensure that you return them to the crib while they feel a bit okay yet awake.

## Growth Spurts

Children grow uniquely from infancy to their teenage years, reaching full physical maturity around 15 to 20 years old. Along the way, they experience sudden growth spurts, marked by rapid increases in height and weight, showcasing their development patterns.

Due to this, your baby may end up sleeping more than usual. This might mean fewer wakeups during the night or longer naps during the day, as their energy goes into the growth process. A small study, as cited by Gates (n.d.-b), indicated that during a growth spurt, babies could end up sleeping up to four and a half hours more than their usual amount over one to two days.

Like physical growth spurts, children also have mental growth spurts. They learn to do things like roll, talk, and crawl. These spurts often happen at the same time as changes in sleep patterns, like around 12 to 19 weeks when they're more cautious with new people or around 13 months when they start worrying when caregivers aren't there.

Neurological changes and mental growth spurts can affect a child's sleep. As their brains develop new skills and connections, sleep disruptions can happen. These changes are part of their progress and learning. Children might cry more, seek more attention and touch, and show crankiness. They could also get frustrated with routines, test boundaries, or become fearful at bedtime. Overall, they might seem fussy during these spurts. Sometimes, if a baby has trouble napping during these times, parents might think about stopping naps or changing bedtime. But it's important not to rush into these decisions too quickly.

During sleep disruptions, it's easy to revert to old habits that can bring back sleep associations. Instead, stick to consistent, independent sleep routines. This is a developmental phase, and normal sleep will return after new skills are learned.

Also, remember that this is a phase of growth, so be patient. Encourage the practice of new skills during the day and promote positive behavior. If disrupted sleep occurs due to growth spurts, try an earlier bedtime to prevent tiredness. Sleep is beneficial for mental growth, helping the brain learn and rest for the next day's activities.

## Developmental Milestones

Whenever your baby learns something new, get ready to feel excited. Sometimes it might not seem like they're changing much, but then suddenly, they'll start showing off how smart they are. Babies who are growing and learning often move forward a bit, but sometimes they also take a small step back.

When babies are getting better at something they're learning, they sometimes have a period of adjustment. They might not feel as calm, wake up more at night, and want more cuddles. Learning new things can be a little scary, so it's normal for babies to want extra comfort from the people they love.

Remember that your child will naturally go through changes as they grow up. These changes are a normal and healthy part of going from a baby to an adult. While you can't control exactly how your child develops, you can control the environment they're in and how you react to them. Be flexible and pay attention to what your baby is telling you.

Don't always assume that changes in your baby's sleep are only because of teething. Sometimes, changes in sleep and how they act are caused by other things. Babies might get used to needing certain things, like being rocked or fed, to fall asleep. Helping your baby sleep better often means teaching them how to soothe themselves.

Give your baby chances to practice new things during the day. Let them spend time on the floor and on their tummies to help them learn to roll over. Try to limit how much time they spend in the stroller or car seat, so they have more chances to practice crawling. Encourage and help your baby as they learn how to control their body.

If your baby gets stuck while trying something, don't rush to help them right away. For example, if they can stand up in their crib but can't get back down, give them time to figure it out. Most new skills have smaller steps, like standing and sitting being different parts.

Learn how to tell when your baby is getting tired. Yawning, rubbing their ears, being fussy, and having trouble focusing are signs that they need sleep. Instead of thinking they need more food or play, understand that these signs mean they're ready for sleep. Babies who aren't sleeping well can become cranky and hard to be around, and they may get really tired.

Every baby grows in their own way and time. Don't worry if your baby's progress is different from another baby's at the same age. Sometimes, babies who take longer to learn something new will catch up later. Just be patient and comforting as your baby learns and grows from trying something new to becoming good at it.

When your baby learns new things, it can make them feel tired. Using their bodies and thinking hard both use up energy. So, don't be surprised if their sleep patterns change along with all the other things happening in their lives.

## *Dealing With Sleep Regressions*

Imagine this: Your baby has been sleeping peacefully, giving you a chance to rest as well. However, all of a sudden, it's as if the sleep routine you've put so much effort into establishing takes an unexpected turn. Your once-reliable sleeper now appears to have turned into a night owl, avoiding peaceful slumber. This is what they call *sleep regression,* a phase that's both fascinating and challenging in your baby's development. It might leave you wondering what happened to those nights of uninterrupted rest you used to enjoy. If this happens to you, you may ask, How can I deal with it?

You may have recently encountered this situation without realizing it's called sleep regression. Before learning about effective coping strategies, it's crucial to recognize the indicators that your baby is going through them (de Bellefonds, 2022).

- Nighttime waking becomes more frequent than usual.

- Your baby encounters difficulty falling asleep during bedtime routines.

- There is an uptick in fussiness and irritability, often during periods when your baby used to be more content.

- Your baby displays a sudden reluctance or resistance to taking naps, which previously was a smoother process.

Understanding and identifying these signs is crucial for you to address sleep regression effectively and provide appropriate support to help your baby navigate through this phase of disrupted sleep patterns.

*Managing Sleep Regression: Effective Tips*

Rest assured; sleep regression is often a temporary phase. Here's how to manage it with your baby:

- Learn your baby's sleep cues, like rubbing their eyes or fussiness, so you can put them to bed before they get too tired.

- Set up a regular bedtime routine, including dinner, bath time, stories, and soothing words.

- Make sure your baby gets enough daytime sleep to avoid nighttime disruptions.

- If your baby wakes up crying, give them a few minutes to settle. If needed, check on them, pat them gently, and use calming words. Avoid practices like rocking or feeding to help them learn to soothe themselves.

- If your baby is four to six months old, consider trying sleep training for at least two weeks.

- Give your baby extra attention during the day and before bedtime to ease any stress they might have.

These steps can help you navigate sleep regression and ensure better rest for both you and your baby.

# Illness and Sleep: When to Adjust Routines and When to Seek Medical Advice

Teething, growth spurts, or reaching developmental milestones may not be the culprits behind your baby's sleep disturbances. Despite your best efforts, your baby continues to be cranky or lack energy. It's conceivable that an underlying factor, such as illness, is influencing their mood and sleep patterns.

Knowing when your baby might be sick is important. The common sign is having a fever, which means the body is fighting an infection. Watch out for changes in how they act, like being sleepier or fussier than usual—these could be signs of illness. For babies under three months old, fever might be a serious sign of infection, so if they have a fever, especially if they're that young, it's important to see a doctor at once to ensure they get the right care.

When your child is ill, make sure they get plenty of rest and sleep. Check on them often and give them extra food or drinks if needed. Sleep helps their bodies heal and fight infections. Giving them more to eat and drink can keep them hydrated, and it's important to keep a close watch if they have a high fever, throw up, or have diarrhea.

When your child starts feeling better, go back to their regular sleep schedule. It might take a day or even two to get naps back on track and to help your baby adjust to not needing that extra nighttime feeding. If the changes only lasted a few days, it should be easy to get back to the usual routine.

Dealing with sleep regression in your baby is a normal part of parenting. While it can be tough, knowing what might trigger it—like growth spurts or new skills—helps you support your little one better. By paying attention to their sleep signals, sticking to a bedtime routine, making sure they nap enough, and trying sleep training if they're ready, you can handle sleep regression more easily. And if your baby gets sick, keeping an eye out for signs like changes in behavior or fever helps you act fast.

Once they're feeling better, getting back to their usual sleep routine will help things go back to normal. With these tips, you'll be better prepared to handle sleep challenges and help your baby grow up healthy and happy.

# Chapter 8:
# Co-Sleeping and Transitioning to Their Own Bed

Despite consistent reminders from experts, such as the American Academy of Pediatrics (2016b), on the risk of co-sleeping, specifically bed-sharing, many parents still break the rule. The number of infant deaths linked to sleep-related issues hasn't improved in recent years. Babies may sleep in the same room as their parents, close to their bed, but on a separate surface made for them. It's best if this arrangement continues for the baby's first year, and at the very least, for the initial 6 months. So, the idea here is *room-sharing* when it comes to co-sleeping.

## The Pros and Cons of Co-Sleeping

Co-sleeping refers to sleeping near your baby, which could be in the same bed or nearby in the same room (known as room-sharing). Co-sleeping is distinct from bed-sharing, *although it might fall under the same category*. While both co-sleeping and bed-sharing have associated drawbacks, they may also provide advantages.

### Co-Sleeping Benefits

McKenna's (2014) important discovery shows that parents act like an *outsourced regulator or jumper cable* for a growing baby. When parents and babies sleep close, their heartbeats, brain activity, sleep patterns, breathing, and other things affect each other. Being close to an adult's body helps the baby stay warm and comfortable. When babies sleep close and cuddle, like in co-sleeping, it helps them breathe regularly, use energy well, grow faster, and feel less stressed. This is the psychological benefit of co-sleeping.

This is evident in the study of Middlemiss et al. (2012) on 25 infants (4–10 months) who were separated for sleep training and found that while the babies became calmer by the third night, their cortisol levels, a stress hormone, remained elevated—meaning they weren't comfortable in their sleep without their mother's presence, especially at the onset of their sleep training.

Babies don't always wake up solely to feed. They might also wake up to seek emotional comfort, and when they're awakened and then comforted by their mothers through touching, hugging, checking, or soothing words, you can observe a range of physiological changes (McKenna, 2014). These include an elevated heart rate and improved oxygen levels as detected by oximetry. The experience is truly remarkable to witness. Therefore, the mother's presence is beneficial during the baby's sleep.

"The different cultures and experiences play a significant role in parent-infant sleep challenges," said McKenna. The safety and benefits of *bed-sharing* can vary based on cultural practices (even though the AAP highly discourages it). McKenna promoted bed-sharing for a specific reason. For example, bed-sharing is common and widely accepted in some contexts, promoting bonding between parents and infants.

However, in other places, safety concerns about bed-sharing may arise due to variations in sleeping arrangements and cultural norms. But if you want to consider bed-sharing, it's important to note that while McKenna provides guidelines for safe bed-sharing, individual instances may vary. You should always consider your situation, be attentive to your baby's needs, and prioritize safety when deciding whether to engage in bed-sharing.

Bed-sharing may result in longer sleep for both adults and babies. You don't need to get up to feed your baby; instead, you can simply lie down on your side and feed your baby while comforting them to sleep. However, safety remains a priority. Make sure that you don't fall asleep while your baby is feeding to prevent any unwanted incidents. Once your baby has finished feeding, transfer them to their crib.

Fathers who bed-share with their babies also experience benefits; a study (Gettler et al., 2012) showed that their testosterone levels decrease more when sleeping close to their babies than those who sleep separately. Bed-sharing children usually start sleeping on their own about a year later, but they often show more self-reliance and confidence in daily life than non-bed-sharing children.

### Co-Sleeping Disadvantages

Every year, about 3500 babies pass away from Sudden Infant Death Syndrome (SIDS), with accidental strangulation and suffocation in bed being a major cause. To keep babies safe while sleeping, the AAP strongly advises following certain guidelines. These include placing babies on their backs on a firm surface without loose clothing, blankets, or soft items nearby. As a new parent, it's important to know and practice safe sleep recommendations.

If you're a mom who stays home or has a long maternity leave, you're probably with your child most of the time. For many moms, the only time they get to be alone is in the evening after the baby is asleep. But if you share a bed with your child, and they need you to fall asleep, this *alone* time won't be experienced anymore.

Further, if you're sharing a bed, you're more likely to fall asleep first, especially when you're tired and alone without someone watching over you and the baby. Instances of strangulation or suffocation might occur, so always remain attentive to your baby.

Refrain from bed-sharing if you smoke, are under the influence of alcohol, or are significantly overweight, and ensure you're on a firm mattress (avoiding waterbeds and couches) while keeping pillows and thick blankets away from the baby.

By adhering to safety practices, co-sleeping may be applied. It's worth noting that it also promotes breastfeeding by maintaining a healthy milk supply through nighttime nursing. Engaging in safe co-sleeping practices can also enhance your sleep quality.

## *When and How to Transition to a Separate Bed*

Both co-sleeping and bed-sharing have been experienced by Alex Mlynek (2012), the mother of a 2-year-old boy who's been sleeping with her. Initially, she hadn't planned on sharing a bed with her 2-year-old son, who used to sleep in his bassinet. However, she decided to try bed-sharing *once* out of exhaustion. Surprisingly, it turned out to be beneficial. She didn't need to get up for nighttime breastfeeding; she experienced longer and better sleep, and her son seemed more comfortable during breastfeeding as well.

While this may sound appealing, planning to transition a child to their own bed can pose a challenge, as they might have become accustomed to bed-sharing or co-sleeping. The question arises: *When and how should you make this transition for your baby?*

Transitioning your baby from co-sleeping or sharing your bed to sleeping on their own is an important step. When to make this change depends on a few things.

- First, think about your baby's age. Usually, around six months old is a good time, as babies have grown and developed enough. But remember, every baby is different.

- Look at how your baby sleeps. If they sleep through the night and have a regular sleep routine, it might be time. But if they still wake up a lot, it could be better to wait.

- Where your baby sleeps matters too. If they've been sleeping with you, start by moving their bed into your room before moving it to their own space. This helps them get used to it.

- Watch how your baby acts. If they're becoming more independent during the day, it might be a sign they're ready to sleep alone at night. But if they get upset when you're not there, they might need more time.

Remember, there's no rush. Take your time and make the transition when your baby is ready. It might take a while, but that's okay. Just be patient and create a comfy sleeping place for them. Slowly getting them used to the idea and giving them comfort will make this change easier for both of you.

To help your baby transition from co-sleeping or sharing your bed to their own, go slowly. Start by making a bedtime routine with calming activities. Put their bed in your room first, and then move it to their space bit by bit. Give them something comforting, like a soft toy, and be there to comfort them if they wake up at night. With time, they'll get used to sleeping on their own.

Brandwein (2022) offers helpful, detailed suggestions to make this transition smoother:

- Gradually use a bedside co-sleeper or bassinet to create more space between you and your child while staying close. This helps both of you adjust to the change.

- Try moving your child's crib into your room temporarily to keep them nearby while transitioning away from bed-sharing. If space is an issue, consider using a bassinet.

- Another option is to sleep temporarily in your child's room, so you're still close during the transition. Keep this arrangement short-term and gradually move away as your child gets used to the new setup.

- Establish a consistent bedtime routine, even while co-sleeping, and make sure to do it in your child's room to create a familiar sleep environment.

- Spend awake time in your child's nursery doing activities like changing diapers, playing, and doing post-bath routines. This helps your child feel comfortable in their sleeping space.

- Start by having your child nap in the crib during the day to help them get used to the new sleeping arrangement. This will make the transition to nighttime sleep easier.

Remember, moving from co-sleeping to the crib is a big change for both you and your child, and it may come with some challenges and emotions.

## *Easing the Transition With Comfort Objects and Routines*

Transitioning your baby to their room or bed can be challenging if they're used to sleeping with you. Here are some suggestions that may help in transitioning your child to their bed from co-sleeping and bed-sharing:

Encourage your child to personalize their new bed with comforting items like soft toys and a special blanket from the cot, and consider adding a night light to ease any fears, such as fear of the dark, in addition to placing additional toys in their bed to provide comfort (Better Health Channel, n.d.)

Donald Winnicott, a respected pediatrician and psychoanalyst, as cited by Lewis (2023), emphasizes that comfort objects play a vital role in reminding children of love and security. These objects, commonly referred to as comfort items, serve to provide infants and children with a sense of solace, promoting feelings of tranquility and safety. Typically held close during bedtime, these items can also offer comfort throughout the day, becoming cherished companions that soothe and reassure.

Toys, often soft, cuddly, and tactilely pleasing, hold a special place in a child's heart, forming a deep emotional connection and aiding in their transition from dependency to self-sufficiency. These transitional objects help children navigate the journey from infancy to early childhood, symbolizing a bridge between the stages. Common examples include soft toys like teddy bears or plushies, comforting blankets such as fluffy covers or baby comforters, and even fragments of a parent's clothing, like a silky tie or a piece of dressing gown trim. Each child may find comfort in different objects, but the underlying principle remains constant: Comfort items serve as steadfast companions that offer solace and a sense of security throughout a child's development.

Please keep in mind that the AAP suggests sharing a room with your baby, as it can lower the risk of SIDS by up to 50% and is significantly safer than sharing a bed. Having your baby in the same room will also simplify feeding, soothing, and keeping an eye on them.

# Chapter 9:
# Sleep for the Breastfeeding Mom

Breastfed babies require feeding every 2–3 hours (8–12 times a day), causing new mothers to miss out on REM sleep. REM sleep begins around 90 minutes into the sleep cycle. Insufficient REM sleep can have an impact on *maternal cognitive function* and *their ability to manage their daily responsibilities*.

If you are a mom, perhaps you've experienced moments when your mind goes blank during the day, you lose focus, and you can't fully attend to your baby's needs. Your sleep could be one factor. Sleep for breastfeeding moms affects their overall wellbeing. If their health is not good, they likely can't produce as much milk as they should, and stress affects it even more. How can you avoid this situation?

## *Managing Sleep While Breastfeeding on Demand*

When mothers breastfeed, they release a natural chemical called oxytocin, otherwise known as love hormones, inducing an emotional connection to their babies, and serving as a natural anxiety relief. Oxytocin has a significant function in fostering attachment between babies and parents through initial contact and interaction during the early stages (Scatliffe et al., 2019). Skin-to-skin contact led to a notable rise in oxytocin levels in infants, mothers, and fathers. Parents with elevated oxytocin levels displayed greater harmony and attentiveness in their interactions with their infants.

To sustain breastfeeding in this regard, you can maintain your sleep by adhering to these measures:

- In the first few weeks, lots of people will want to visit and celebrate with you and the new baby. But it's a good idea to limit visitors during this time. This is when you and your baby need to spend time together, healing, resting, and sleeping.

- Learn how to comfortably nurse while lying on your side. This is a safe and effective way for you and your baby to rest while breastfeeding during the day. You can rest here, but *don't* sleep to avoid untoward incidents. Resting may help relax the body for a while.

- Taking a nap is a great way to make up for the sleep you lost during the night. You might have heard the phrase *sleep when the baby sleeps*, and though it's not always easy, it's worth trying. If possible, have someone at home who can help with cooking, cleaning, and laundry, as this may let you focus on yourself and your baby, so you can get some extra sleep.

- Put your baby to sleep in a crib next to your bed. This will prevent you from having to go back and forth to the nursery and will give you a chance to get more sleep. Also, if you have previously breastfed your baby on the bed while lying on your side, you may want to put your baby back in the crib once they're feeling drowsy. This way, you can also sleep well in your bed without thinking so much.

- Don't watch your clock to check what time it is. "Observing the time on the clock can lead to anxiety about not being able to return to sleep," said Dr. Brian Murray, as cited by Romero (2023), a sleep neurologist at Sunnybrook Health Sciences Centre in Toronto, Canada, during a 2016 interview with CBC News. "It triggers the body to release fight-or-flight hormones, which disrupt the process of falling asleep."

Don't hesitate to ask for help from your loved ones. Getting help with everyday tasks, even simple ones like laundry and dishes, gives you time to rest and do things that help you feel better emotionally.

## *Pumping and Storing Milk for Nighttime Feedings*

Whether you're resuming work (either day or night shifts), ask your partner to assist with feeding, and ensure a supply of breastmilk for your baby during your brief absence. You'll also need proper guidance on effectively pumping and safely storing your breastmilk.

### *Pumping*

When preparing to pump, ensure cleanliness by washing your hands with soap and water or using an alcohol-based hand sanitizer. Also, maintain a clean pumping area, including pump parts and bottles, while you don't need to wash your breasts and nipples beforehand.

To help stimulate milk flow without your baby, you can utilize techniques such as reflecting on your baby's positive aspects, having their photo or scented item nearby, applying a warm cloth to your breasts, gently massaging your breasts and nipples, imagining the milk flow, and finding a peaceful place to relax. Employing these strategies can lead to a smoother and more comfortable pumping experience.

It's crucial to note that supplying breast milk using a pump or by hand can be achieved through three methods: hand pumping, electric pumping, and manually operated pumping (Office on Women's Health, 2017).

- **Hand pumping**. You employ your hand to gently squeeze and apply pressure to your breast to express milk.

- **Electric pumping**. An electric pump operates using either a battery or by connecting to an electrical socket.

- **Manually operated pumping**. You employ your hand and wrist to operate a handheld device designed for milk pumping.

You have the option to borrow an electric pump from a lactation specialist at a nearby hospital or through a breastfeeding group. This variety of pumps is effective for establishing milk production when direct breastfeeding isn't possible for a new baby. Mothers who faced challenges with different pumping techniques might discover these pumps to be particularly beneficial for their needs.

### *Storing*

Understanding how to feed your baby is essential, but proper milk storage is just as vital. And when I mention storage, it's not about placing it anywhere, anytime. You also need to contemplate where, when, and for how long it should be stored. Here are the tips (CDC, 2020):

- Put a clear date label on your breast milk.

- No fridge or freezer door storage: This prevents temperature fluctuations caused by frequent opening and closing of the door.

- If you won't use fresh milk in four days, freeze it immediately. That keeps the milk quality top-notch. Freshly expressed breast milk can be stored in the refrigerator for a maximum of four days. It is recommended to keep the breast milk within a temperature range of 32°F to 39°F (0°C to 4°C) for optimal storage.

- Freezing milk? Keep it small—store two to four ounces, or what's needed for one feeding.

- Mark the container with the child's name if you're handing it over to childcare. And chat with them about other labeling and storage needs.

- Traveling? Chill with ice packs for 24 hours in an insulated cooler. Once you land, use it, pop it in the fridge, or freeze it.

Once breast milk is thawed, it should be used within 24 hours to maintain its nutritional quality. The CDC advises against refreezing thawed milk, as it can negatively impact the milk's composition and safety. If you do so, it should only be stored for up to one day in the refrigerator.

## *Strategies for Getting Enough Rest as a Breastfeeding Mother*

Sleep deprivation is common when you're a new parent. Breastfeeding, just like preparing a formula bottle, can disrupt sleep. However, following some suggested strategies by Stone (2013) can assist you in getting enough rest:

- **Breastfeed more often during the day**. Offer the breast regularly while awake to potentially reduce nighttime waking and stimulate milk supply. Working moms can pump more frequently, too.

- **Keep the baby close in the evening**. Have the baby nearby in a sling or on your lap during quiet evening activities to encourage cluster feeding.

- **Feed the baby before bedtime**. Wake baby for a nursing session before you go to sleep to ensure a full tummy and leverage sleep-inducing hormones.

- **Consider safe co-sleeping**. Keep the baby nearby to tend to their needs without fully waking up but be cautious and prepared for intentional co-sleeping.

- **Arrange daytime help**. When babies can't go without nursing, have someone you trust take them for a walk or look after them so you can nap or rest.

Finding a good balance between breastfeeding and helping your baby sleep well is really important for moms. It means feeding your baby more during the day to possibly reduce nighttime wakeups, considering safe ways to sleep together, and getting help for daytime naps. By trying out these ideas and adjusting them to your situation, you can make sure your baby gets enough food and sleep, which makes being a parent easier and more satisfying.

# Chapter 10:
# Sibling Sleep Dynamics

Bedtime becomes a playground for bonding and connections between brothers and sisters. Imagine the joy of hushed laughter, the thrill of whispered secrets, and the occasional tug-of-war over blankets. Have you ever wondered how these bedtime interactions influence the relationships and sleep patterns of siblings? How can you ensure your kids sleep well while nurturing their sibling bonds?

## *Encouraging Healthy Sleep Habits for Older Siblings*

Children's sleep is influenced by their environment and genes. Family stress and conflicts can affect sleep, but it's unclear if sibling fights impact sleep too. Breitenstein et al., (2018) studied 582 twins and found that more sibling conflict was linked to shorter sleep and more sleep problems, even when considering other factors like stress at home. Genes play a bigger role in sleep duration as they grow older. These findings suggest that helping parents improve sibling relationships and sleep habits could make a positive difference.

Naturally, sibling conflicts arise, especially when they're close in age or due to clashes of personalities. Even if there isn't any overt conflict, and they get along like best friends, they might end up playing all night instead of sleeping. This presents a challenge that parents need to address and manage.

The initial step for parents is to align their children's ages and personalities. Lauren Gardner, Ph.D., ABPP, who serves as the Psychology Internship Director and Administrative Director of the Autism Program at Johns Hopkins All Children's Hospital, suggests that closely matching children by age enables them to be more compatible roommates. She also noted that when siblings are of similar ages and developmental stages, parents can often coordinate their schedules to align bedtimes. This synchronization can make the bedtime routine more efficient and potentially contribute to improved sleep for both children, as reported by Fleming (2022).

Another issue arises when their sleep gets disturbed due to the needs of their younger siblings. This doesn't just affect the parents' sleep; at times, it also affects the sleep of the older siblings. In this case, try your best to stick to the bedtime routine that your older child is used to. Also, try to do this routine with just your older child, without their younger sibling. This will give your older child special time that they'll like, and it can also stop them from feeling jealous of their sibling. Because babies usually go to sleep later than older kids, it might be tough for your older child to see the baby getting attention from mom or dad while they have to stay in bed (LoMonaco, 2023).

Another crucial aspect of practicing good sleep habits involves creating a suitable sleeping environment in the bedroom. The room should be dimly lit and free from excessive distractions. Bedrooms with bright alarm clocks, blinking lights from gaming consoles, and phones vibrating with incoming messages can potentially disrupt children's sleep routines. To encourage improved sleep, it's beneficial to have bedrooms that aren't overly warm and feel comfortable. While some kids enjoy sleeping with heavy blankets, they might end up feeling too hot and uncomfortable. Try using thinner blankets and lighter pajamas.

The hardest part of getting kids to sleep is when parents don't do the same things every time. Once you have a plan, stick to it. Be like a clock that always does the same things at the same time. For example, if you plan to take a bath, read a story, and then turn off the lights, your child should know that's what will happen. This makes them feel calm, and they have time to get sleepy before it's suddenly time to sleep. Hence, consistency is the key—continue doing the usual routine.

## *Navigating Shared Bedrooms and Sleep Routines*

Sharing a sleeping space can disrupt siblings' sleep due to physical disturbances, differing sleep patterns, and potential psychological effects like delayed sleep onset and heightened excitement. When dealing with shared bedrooms and sleep routines for older siblings, there are a few things to consider:

- **Keep up the usual routine**. It's a good idea to create a bedtime routine that works for both of them. This routine should help them relax and get ready for sleep.

- **Separate siblings**. If you can, try to give each sibling their own space within the shared room. This can be done with things like curtains or dividers. It's important for them to feel like they have their place. It's important to note that siblings under the age of one should not sleep together in the same bed (Willes, 2017).

- **Sleep at the same time**. If possible, have them go to bed around the same time. This way, they won't bother each other when one wants to sleep and the other wants to be awake.

- **Avoid any noise**. Noise can be a problem in shared rooms. To fix this, you can use things like white noise machines or soft music to cover up sounds that might wake one sibling while the other is still awake.

- **Have a personal talk**. Talk to your older kids about how they like to sleep and any issues they have. This way, they can be part of finding solutions.

- **Let them decide on their own**. As they grow up, let them do more things on their own when it comes to bedtime. This can help them feel responsible.

- **Involve your kids in decision-making**. If there are arguments or problems, involve your older kids in finding solutions together. Teach them about working together and thinking about each other's needs.

- **Monitor their sleep habits**. Keep an eye on how things are going. If there are ongoing problems, be ready to change things to make them work better.

Overall, creating a peaceful sleep situation for older siblings and sharing a room involves talking openly, being flexible, and finding ways to make each child comfortable and happy.

## *Strategies for Minimizing Sleep Disruptions Between Siblings*

Owens (2020) explored sleep disturbances, identifying two categories of factors: intrinsic and extrinsic. Intrinsic factors encompass emotional and psychological aspects, while extrinsic factors are environmental. One such environmental factor is housing arrangements that necessitate siblings sharing a room. Supporting this, Willes (2017) highlighted that when younger siblings share a room with toddlers, scenarios like playing with toys or unintentionally waking their sleeping sibling can lead to disruptions.

The sleep of siblings, particularly those of the same age or twins, can be significantly impacted by engaging in pre-bedtime activities together. This interaction can lead to disruptions in their sleep patterns. These disruptions can manifest in various ways. To address this, it's important to consider strategies that mitigate these disruptions and foster improved sleep quality for both siblings. What specific sleep disturbances might arise, and how can you effectively minimize them to encourage better sleep? Willes (2017) shared her tips for twins that also work well for siblings close in age who are sharing a room.

- Choose a primary baby, usually the one who cries more than their sibling. Time intervals and feedings (if applicable) will be based on this baby. For example, if the primary baby cries continuously for 10 minutes while the other cries on and off, check on both babies at the same time. If the primary baby wakes up at 1:30 a.m. for a feed, wake and feed the sibling as well. Remember, it's not necessary to check on both babies during every visit. If the calmer child is almost asleep while the other has been crying for 10 minutes, you can leave the calmer one and focus on the crying child during the check.

- Alternatively, you can separately train your children, even if they share a room. This approach is smoother with two adults involved. Each baby has their own time and a designated caretaker. For instance, if child A is with mom and child B is with dad, dad sets the timer and attends to child B only (as mom is tending to child A). This method works best when babies are too young to notice when one parent enters and exits the room without interacting with them. This is apart from using white noise machines, dim lights, keeping a usual routine, and so on.

Getting good sleep is important for siblings who share a room. Sleep helps kids grow, think, feel happy, and stay healthy. When siblings share a room, how they sleep and the things around them can affect each other's sleep. This means if one sibling has trouble sleeping, it might affect the other one too. So, making sure both siblings have a comfy sleep space and a regular sleep routine is helpful for them to sleep well.

# Chapter 11: Travel and Sleep

There inevitably comes a moment when families need to escape the hustle and bustle of city life to unwind in a new setting. Family trips and vacations have become commonplace as opportunities for bonding and relaxation in today's fast-paced world. However, when children are young, maintaining their sleep schedules can be tricky due to factors like varying time zones. If you're preparing to travel with your children, adhering to some guidelines for managing sleep routines could prove beneficial.

## *Tips for Managing Sleep Routines While Traveling*

Balancing sleep routines during travel poses a challenge for parents, particularly when embarking on family trips for the first time. Sleep routines, encompassing schedules, surroundings, and sleeping arrangements, can be disrupted due to varying time zones and new environments. Here are some strategies to help you navigate this situation (Mitchell, n.d.):

• Allow your baby to sleep the way they do when they're at home. If they sleep in the same room as you at home, continue that arrangement during your vacation. If they have their own sleeping area at home, try to provide a similar space for them during the trip, if feasible.

• Bring the things that remind them of home, like their sleep sack, favorite cuddly item, and lullabies.

• Try to follow your nap schedule as much as possible, but if it doesn't go as planned, don't worry too much. Remember to enjoy your vacation, as nothing has to be flawless. But if your baby wants to nap, let them be. The longer the nap, the better.

• If your baby falls asleep while moving or while you're out, try to keep the motion going so they can have a nap of at least 45 minutes or longer.

• To ensure better sleep for your child, it's important to maintain your regular bedtime routine and be consistent in how you respond to nighttime waking. These actions help establish a predictable sleep pattern and create a sense of security, promoting more restful nights.

## *Managing Time Zone Changes and Jet Lag*

Jet lag can mess up a baby's sleep because the time changes can confuse their internal body clock. The effort you put in previously to align the proper sleep schedule for your baby (circadian rhythm) will come into play again. However, there's no need to be concerned. You can make things right again with the recommendations provided by Iturmendi (2018) and BabySleepCode (2022).

• **Adjust to a new time zone starting at home**. According to Iturmendi, getting a head start by slowly changing your baby's schedule a few days before the flight is a smart move. Depending on your destination, you can shift bedtime a bit later or earlier and align naps accordingly. This approach also applies to waking up in the morning. By doing this, your baby's body will handle time changes with less difficulty.

• **Adjust to the current time zone while in the destination**. Try to match your baby's naps with the new time and help them stay awake a little longer if needed, especially by playing outside. Sunlight is really helpful. Keep your baby active during the day, and when it's time to sleep, make the room cozy with soft lighting and quiet talk. You can also help your baby sleep by giving them a warm bath, reading a story, or singing a lullaby.

- **Rest when your baby rests**. There's not much more to include on this topic. The guideline remains quite similar to when your baby was born. As jet lag affects you as well, it's crucial to make the most of your *time off.*

- **Handle nighttime awakenings**. Your baby might wake up during the night. To handle this, aim for a calm approach: use soft lights, speak gently, and avoid playful activities. If your baby doesn't usually eat at night, try to limit nighttime feedings. If your baby wakes up late at night and is content in their crib, it's okay to leave them. On the flip side, if they're wide awake and want to get up, don't worry too much about trying to settle them down at once. Allowing them a short period of wakefulness can help rebuild their need for sleep. Just watch for signs of tiredness and gently put them back in their crib when they're ready to fall asleep.

- **Understand differing sleep patterns**. It's alright if your baby goes to sleep earlier than usual. Aim for a somewhat reasonable bedtime without making them overly tired. Remember, if they fall asleep around 5 p.m., they might wake up as early as 5 a.m. the next day. So, be prepared for an early start.

Try to keep your usual bedtime routine intact to help your child settle down comfortably. Use the familiar sleep cues you use at home to make them feel at ease in the new place.

## *Creating a Portable Sleep-Friendly Environment*

Who would prefer to have their baby constantly in their arms during a trip? Instead of enjoying the opportunity to explore, you might end up cutting your outing short due to fatigue from holding your baby. Many parents aim for their kids to feel secure and cozy when traveling, yet finding the right bed can feel overwhelming. Luckily, there are numerous choices suggested by Gallo (2023) that can enhance your travel experience with your little one, making it more pleasant and comfortable.

- **Travel tents**. If you're planning a camping or beach trip with your toddler, a travel tent could be a useful option. While there have been concerns about entrapment risks and suffocation associated with travel tents (Swartz, 2012), they can still be suitable for toddlers aged 1 and older (not recommended under 1 year of age). Various brands offer travel tents but prioritize choosing one that has a proven safety record for children.

- **Travel cribs**. Travel cribs are a smart choice for trips with kids since numerous accommodations might not be child friendly. These cribs aren't only useful for travel; they can also serve a dual purpose at home.

- **Inflatable beds**. Top-notch inflatable toddler beds are carefully designed. They come with a removable internal mattress that makes it simple to put on sheets. These beds feature bumpers to prevent active toddlers from rolling out, and they're covered in soft flocking to provide added comfort.

- **Toddler hammock**. A toddler hammock offers a distinctive and comfy sleep option for parents aiming to give their children a snug and safe sleeping space. Top-notch hammocks are made to be light and simple to assemble, constructed from strong materials, and can hold a toddler's weight. Plus, many toddler hammocks include a carry bag for convenient transportation.

- **Toddler sleeping bag**. This offers an easy and budget-friendly sleeping option for parents going camping or glamping with their young children. It's made to keep kids warm and cozy, and it's great for camping trips or sleepovers. Many safe toddler sleeping bags even have a built-in pillow and can be conveniently rolled up and stored in a carry bag. They're lightweight too, allowing you to carry them on your back, which is perfect for hiking and outdoor adventures.

When purchasing a travel bed, it's crucial to thoroughly assess the company's credibility and research any instances of entrapment or suffocation that have been reported. Opt for a high-quality bed that is suitable for your child's age. If you plan to place your infant on the portable bed, ensure that you closely supervise them and stay right next to them.

# Chapter 12:
# Long-Term Solutions

Although welcoming a baby brings excitement, it also comes with difficulties. Nurturing little ones is a demanding task, especially during the initial period when tiredness and lack of sleep can be overwhelming. But don't fret! This phase of sleeplessness is temporary. As they grow older, their sleep changes as well—they'll sleep more at night and only have one nap a day. And you'll slowly recover your long, wanted sleep.

## *Adapting Sleep Routines as Your Child Grows*

The phases from being a newborn to becoming a toddler can prove to be the most challenging, especially when you're yearning for a tranquil night's sleep. Applying the method and the suggestions from the sleep experts stated previously may help you adjust to sleep routines as your child grows. Always keep in mind the following when your child is (LoRe, 2023):

**a newborn**

- Enhance your baby's bedtime routine and promote better sleep for your newborn with these valuable tips: Prevent overtiredness by managing sleep timing while also creating a soothing sleep environment. Swaddling can provide comfort and maintaining a cool room temperature aids sleep quality. Quick nighttime diaper changes and sharing bedtime responsibilities with your partner can help optimize the routine. Consider using a pacifier if suitable and remain adaptable to nap variations. Establish a consistent bedtime routine and exercise patience and consistency throughout the process.

**six months or older**

- **Establish a regular routine for bedtime**. If you haven't already, it's a great idea to create a bedtime routine for your little one. Think of it as a special signal to your child that it's time to wind down and go to sleep. Consistently following this routine can improve your baby's sleep and bring more harmony to your family's daily routine. This effort will pay off.

- **Follow the right schedule for their age**. Overly tired babies might fuss more before bedtime and have less restful sleep. On the other hand, babies who aren't tired enough might struggle to fall asleep due to insufficient sleep pressure. Finding the ideal bedtime helps with sleep training and makes things smoother.

- **Break sleep training into steps**. When addressing sleep issues during both the day and night, it can be tempting to tackle everything at once. However, this approach can lead to overwhelm and increased fussiness. Instead, approach it in stages. Start with bedtime, as mastering this often reduces nighttime waking. Once bedtime is successful, focus on naps. Although it may take more time, this method keeps things manageable and promotes consistency.

- **Stay committed**. Teaching healthy sleep habits is a long-term commitment. After your baby learns to fall asleep on their own, it's important to continue supporting them to maintain their sleep patterns. It's okay to occasionally rock or feed them to sleep, especially when they're unwell or during vacations. Just remember that this might temporarily affect their progress.

When picking a sleep training method for your baby, it's a good idea to consider the suggestions given. Just make sure to follow advice from sleep experts, like the ones mentioned earlier.

## *Encouraging Independent Sleep Skills*

Encouraging independent sleep in babies involves establishing a consistent routine. Start with a calming, pre-sleep ritual to signal bedtime, such as a warm bath, gentle rocking, or reading a story. Ensure the sleep environment is cozy and soothing by dimming the lights, keeping the room quiet, and maintaining a comfortable temperature. Place your baby in their crib while they are drowsy but still awake to help them learn how to soothe themselves to sleep. This step helps them associate their crib with sleep and enables them to fall asleep independently.

As your baby grows, practice allowing them some time to settle on their own if they wake up during the night. Not rushing in at every little sound gives them a chance to learn how to self-soothe back to sleep. It's important to be patient and consistent with these practices, as it might take time for your baby to fully adjust to sleeping independently. Over time, these efforts can foster healthy sleep habits and help your baby become more confident in falling and staying asleep on their own.

Another suggestion from The Children's Hospital of Philadelphia (2014) may also help to encourage your baby to sleep on their own:

- **Stay active throughout the day**. A well-exercised baby sleeps more soundly. Ensure your baby has playtime between naps, encouraging them to crawl, cruise, bounce, and giggle.

- **Avoid rocking**. Don't wait until your baby is asleep before placing them in their crib. If you always rock them to sleep, or they rely on feeding to doze off, they may struggle to sleep independently. Put your baby in their crib, both for naps and bedtime, when they're drowsy but still awake.

- **Allow gentle fussing**. When your baby starts fussing, give them some space. Let them try to fall asleep on their own. If their crying persists for a few minutes, you can go into their room. Keep the room dim and refrain from picking them up or playing. Offer a gentle pat on their tummy and softly tell them to go back to sleep. If they have a pacifier, you can give it back to them, speaking in a soothing and calm tone.

- **Stay patient**. It may take a few weeks for your baby to learn how to self-soothe and return to sleep on their own. Stay committed, and eventually, you'll all enjoy peaceful nights.

## *Preparing for the Transition From Crib to Toddler Bed*

As your child grows into a toddler, there will come a point when they need their own space to foster independence and responsibility. Preparing for the transition from a crib to a toddler bed is a significant milestone. Here's how you can make it go smoothly:

- **Choose the right time**. Think about when your child is ready. Most kids transition between 1.5 and 3 years old, but each child is different. Look for signs such as climbing out of the crib or showing interest in a big kid bed.

- **Include them**. Make it exciting by involving your child in the decision-making process. They can participate in selecting their new bed or choosing special bedding, which will generate excitement and make them feel more involved in the change.

- **Safety first**. Make sure the new bed is safe. Utilize safety rails to prevent falling. Ensure that any furniture is properly secured to prevent tipping. Maintain a room free from any potential hazards.

- **Keep things familiar**. Use the same items from their crib, such as blankets and stuffed animals, to make the new bed feel cozy and familiar.

- **Keep a routine**. Stick to a consistent bedtime routine. This helps children understand that it's time to unwind and sleep, similar to when they were in the crib.

- **Say good things**. Praise them for their successful adaptation and create a joyful atmosphere by discussing the exciting activities they can enjoy in their new bed.

- **Safety rules**. Teach them about staying safe in their new bed, including showing them where the edges are and explaining the importance of staying in bed at night.

- **Take small steps**. If possible, begin by using the new bed for naps. This will help them acclimate to it before sleeping there at night.

- **Stay nearby**. Be prepared for them to rise from bed initially. Carefully guide them back without making it a significant issue.

- **Keep going**. Be patient and continue with the same routine each night. It may take a few nights for them to feel comfortable in the new bed.

Remember, every child is unique. Some may embrace the new bed immediately, while others may require additional time. Offer your support and encouragement throughout this exciting transition.

Modifying sleep routines for infants, promoting independent sleep, and transitioning them from cribs to beds are crucial for their development. These practices help them learn self-soothing techniques, build confidence, and achieve important milestones. By approaching these changes with patience and consistency, you establish a solid foundation for healthy sleep.

# Conclusion

*Motherhood: the days are long, but the years are short.* –Gretchen Rubin

Let's talk about Elaine Jacobson again. Do you remember her? I shared her story at the beginning of this parenting journey. You may be wondering how things turned out for her. The good news is that she did recover. She only needed strong medication for a year. She went through a tough time with postpartum depression, which she didn't even realize she had until after her second child was born. But with the help of her doctor, Dr. Santiago-Munoz, she started feeling better and happier.

Postpartum depression is a real thing! While some people might say it's all in your head, it's a very real struggle for certain moms, especially those without enough support, proper food, or good sleep. People don't always realize how important sleep is. When moms don't get enough sleep, they can't focus properly, and that might lead to accidents that affect their babies. And even babies who don't get enough attention can have problems, like not eating well or having trouble sleeping.

Sleep is just as important as eating and drinking water, not only for babies but for everyone. To all the strong moms out there who become even stronger for their kids, you're the real heroes! You have this natural ability to take care of your children without expecting anything back. Everyone loves you for it!

If you want to take good care of your baby, you also need to take good care of yourself. Your health affects your baby's health as well. Get enough sleep and eat well so you can take care of your kids and your whole family!

When I had my first baby, it felt like riding a roller coaster. I had to juggle my job and take care of my child all at once. Those first few weeks were tough. My whole body hurt, and I had to feed my baby every 2–3 hours, even at night. It got even harder when I couldn't breastfeed anymore, so I had to use formula. I went for three months without proper sleep because I had to prepare formula whenever my baby woke up at night. It was challenging, working during the day and relying on my family's help when I wasn't there. I'm grateful for their support.

Now that my son is older, I get better sleep, and he's growing up healthy, even though he's on formula. As long as formula-fed babies are well taken care of, they can be just as happy and healthy. I have no regrets about those tough times. They helped me understand the struggles mothers face, especially my mother. I also learned the importance of sleep, whether I have kids or not. The most crucial moments for children's development are during those early months, which I've come to realize. They become smarter, healthier, and better behaved when they're loved and cared for from the moment they're born up to this day.

So, to all the moms out there, whether you're new to this or you've been through it before, take it easy. Relax. If your baby is sleeping, take advantage of that time. They won't be babies forever, and sooner than you think, they'll grow up so fast. You'll miss their chubby cheeks when they're around 4–6 months old. The first words and smiles they have in those initial months will become cherished memories. One day, they will leave home and embark on their own journey, just as you did with your parents.

While they're still little, seize the moments, even if you're not getting enough sleep. They won't be this young for long. And remember, if you want to make things a bit easier as a new parent, you can try using sleep training methods and following suggestions to help both you and your baby sleep better. Sleep is vital for their growth; it's when they process what they've learned, embrace new experiences, and wake up ready to learn even more with you in every stage of their development.

I'm a mom who has read books about babies, their sleep needs, and everything in between. Drawing from my experience as a mother, I believe it's valuable to share my struggles and the lessons I've learned throughout my journey of parenthood, from newborn to toddler to teen. It's not an easy path, but you'll come to understand the importance of patience, practicality, resourcefulness, care, and love. Having your own baby will also help you discover more about yourself—at least, that's what I've personally experienced. That goes for babies everywhere, *Sweet Dreams*!

# References


Abbott, R. C. (2021, March 8). *Does Culture Impact How A Baby Sleeps?* Childhood & Education. https://medium.com/childhood-education/does-culture-impact-how-a-baby-sleeps-cfabe0a50be6

Abdul Jafar, N. K., Tham, E. K. H., Pang, W. W., Fok, D., Chua, M. C., Teoh, O.-H., Goh, D. Y. T., Shek, L. P-C., Yap, F., Tan, K. H., Gluckman, P. D., Chong, Y.-S., Meaney, M. J., Broekman, B. F. P., & Cai, S. (2021). Association between breastfeeding and sleep patterns in infants and preschool children. *The American Journal of Clinical Nutrition.* https://doi.org/10.1093/ajcn/nqab297

Adair, L. (2023, July 3). *How does your parenting style affect sleep coaching?* Lullabies. https://lullabies.ae/post/how-does-your-parenting-style-affect-sleep-coaching

Allen, S. L., Howlett, M. D., Coulombe, J. A., & Corkum, P. V. (2016). ABCs of SLEEPING: A review of the evidence behind pediatric sleep practice recommendations. *Sleep Medicine Reviews, 29,* 1–14. https://doi.org/10.1016/j.smrv.2015.08.006

American Academy of Pediatrics. (2016a). *How to Calm a Fussy Baby: Tips for Parents & Caregivers.* HealthyChildren.org. https://www.healthychildren.org/English/ages-stages/baby/crying-colic/Pages/Calming-A-Fussy-Baby.aspx

American Academy of Pediatrics. (2016b). SIDS and Other Sleep-Related Infant Deaths: Updated 2016 Recommendations for a Safe Infant Sleeping Environment. *Pediatrics, 138*(5), e20162938. https://doi.org/10.1542/peds.2016-2938

American Academy of Pediatrics. (2022, June 21). *American Academy of Pediatrics Updates Safe Sleep Recommendations: Back is Best.* https://www.aap.org/en/news-room/news-releases/aap/2022/american-academy-of-pediatrics-updates-safe-sleep-recommendations-back-is-best/

American Optometric Association. (n.d.). *Infant Vision: Birth to 24 Months of Age.* https://www.aoa.org/healthy-eyes/eye-health-for-life/infant-vision

*Baby care—moving from cot to bed.* (n.d.). Better Health. Retrieved August 18, 2023, from https://www.betterhealth.vic.gov.au/health/healthyliving/baby-care-moving-from-cot-to-bed

BabySleepCode. (2022, November 26). *Navigating baby sleep and jet lag when traveling across time zones.* https://babysleepcode.com.au/blogs/sleep-tips/navigating-baby-sleep-and-jet-lag

*Baby Sleep Training: The Weissbluth Method.* (2012). Education.com. https://www.education.com/magazine/article/weissbluth-method/

Barry, J. (2021, April 28). *How baby milestones affect sleep.* https://www.kidspot.com.au/baby/baby-care/how-baby-milestones-affect-sleep/news-story/f54c6fa3fd3f9c4ef584c45ecd66b348

Berry, J. (2019, December 19). *How to burp a sleeping baby: Effective methods.* Medical News Today. https://www.medicalnewstoday.com/articles/how-to-burp-a-sleeping-baby#what-if-they-dont-burp

Betts, J. L. (2022). *52 Bittersweet Quotes About Children Growing Up Way Too Fast.* LoveToKnow. https://www.lovetoknow.com/quotes-quips/relationships/52-bittersweet-quotes-about-children-growing-up-way-too-fast

Blau, M. (n.d.). *Author*. Retrieved August 16, 2023, from https://melindablau.com/

Brandwein, S. (2020, September 29). *How to Make a Smooth Transition From Co-Sleeping to Crib*. Moshi Kids. https://www.moshikids.com/articles/transition-from-co-sleeping-to-crib/

Breitenstein, R. S., Doane, L. D., Clifford, S., & Lemery-Chalfant, K. (2018). Children's sleep and daytime functioning: Increasing heritability and environmental associations with sibling conflict. *Social Development (Oxford, England)*, *27*(4), 967–983. https://doi.org/10.1111/sode.12302

Brewer, C. (2023, June 19). *13 Best Travel Beds for Toddlers for 2023*. Baby Can Travel. https://www.babycantravel.com/best-toddler-travel-bed/

Brown, A., & Harries, V. (2015). Infant Sleep and Night Feeding Patterns During Later Infancy: Association with Breastfeeding Frequency, Daytime Complementary Food Intake, and Infant Weight. *Breastfeeding Medicine*, *10*(5), 246–252. https://doi.org/10.1089/bfm.2014.0153

Canadian Paediatric Society. (2004). Creating a safe sleep environment for your baby. *Paediatrics & Child Health*, *9*(9), 665–666. https://doi.org/10.1093/pch/9.9.665

CDC. (n.d.). *Human Milk Storage Guidelines STORAGE LOCATIONS AND TEMPERATURES*. Retrieved August 19, 2023, from https://www.cdc.gov/breastfeeding/pdf/HumanMilk-en-5x7-508.pdf

CDC. (2019). *About 3,500 babies in the US are lost to sleep-related deaths each year*. https://www.cdc.gov/media/releases/2018/p0109-sleep-related-deaths.html

CDC. (2020). *Proper Storage and Preparation of Breast Milk*. https://www.cdc.gov/breastfeeding/recommendations/handling_breastmilk.htm

Chapell, M., Sullivan, B., Saridakis, S., Costello, L., Mazgajiewski, N., McGinley, J., McGlone, J., & Pasquarella, A. (2001). Myopia and Night-Time Lighting during Sleep in Children and Adults. *Perceptual and Motor Skills*, *92*(3), 640–642E. https://doi.org/10.2466/pms.2001.92.3.640

Children's Hospital Los Angeles. (2020, July 10). *Your Infant is Teething: Know the Signs and Symptoms*. https://www.chla.org/blog/advice-experts/your-infant-teething-know-signs-and-symptoms

Children's Health of Orange County. (2021, September 27). *Babies and sleep: The ultimate guide*. Children's Health Hub. https://health.choc.org/babies-and-sleep-the-ultimate-guide/

Children's Hospital of Philadelphia. (2014, March 15). *Silent Nights: Helping Your Baby Fall Asleep Independently*. https://www.chop.edu/news/silent-nights-helping-your-baby-fall-asleep-independently

*Choosing a Safe Crib and Bedding*. (2019, August 5). Pediatrics West. https://www.pediatricswest.org/parent-resources/blog/choosing-a-safe-crib-and-bedding/

Cleveland Clinic. (2022, August 23). *6 Bedtime Tips for Babies*. https://health.clevelandclinic.org/bedtime-routine-for-babies/

Contributors, W. E. (2023). *What's the Right Room Temperature for a Baby?* WebMD. https://www.webmd.com/baby/what-is-the-right-room-temperature-for-a-baby

Crider, C. (2019, November 22). *Self-Soothing Baby: Techniques for Helping Baby Settle*. Healthline. https://www.healthline.com/health/baby/self-soothing-baby#know-when-to-start

Dallas Sleep. (n.d.). *The Importance Of Sleep As A New Parent: Dallas Sleep: Snoring & Sleep Apnea Specialists*. Retrieved August 10, 2023, from https://www.dallas-sleep.com/blog/the-importance-of-sleep-as-a-new-parent

de Bellefonds, C. (2022, January 20). *Is Your Baby Going Through a Sleep Regression?* What to Expect. https://www.whattoexpect.com/first-year/sleep/sleep-regression/

Decker, E. (2022, December 8). *Pacifiers: When to Stop Using Them*. Nationwide Childrens. https://www.nationwidechildrens.org/family-resources-education/700childrens/2022/12/pacifiers

Dewar, G. (2018, January 2). *Baby sleep patterns: An evidence-based guide*. PARENTING SCIENCE. https://parentingscience.com/baby-sleep-patterns/

Dewar, G. (2022, July 20). *Dream feeding: An evidence-based guide*. PARENTING SCIENCE. https://parentingscience.com/dream-feeding/

Divecha, D. (2020, February 7). *How Co-sleeping Can Help You and Your Baby*. Berkley. https://greatergood.berkeley.edu/article/item/how_cosleeping_can_help_you_and_your_baby

*Don't look at the clock! And 7 other tips to beat dreaded insomnia*. (2016, July 21). CBC News. https://www.cbc.ca/news/health/insomnia-tips-sleep-1.3677363

Encyclopedia. (n.d.). *Ferber, Richard 1944- (Richard A. Ferber)*. Retrieved August 16, 2023, from https://www.encyclopedia.com/arts/educational-magazines/ferber-richard-1944-richard-ferber

Felson, S. (2005, April 26). *What Are REM and Non-REM Sleep?* WebMD. https://www.webmd.com/sleep-disorders/sleep-101

Fleming, L. (2022). *Handling Bedtimes When Kids Share a Room*. Verywell Family. https://www.verywellfamily.com/dealing-with-bedtimes-when-your-kids-share-a-room-5218951

French, M. (2021, August 28). *Pros & Cons of Co-Sleeping and Bed-Sharing*. BabyQuip. https://www.babyquip.com/blog/co-sleeping-and-bed-sharing#The_Cons

Gagne, C. (2021, April 2). *How to stop co-sleeping: An age-by-age guide*. Todays Parent. https://www.todaysparent.com/family/family-health/how-to-stop-co-sleeping-an-age-by-age-guide/

Gallo, A. (2023, March 22). *Best Travel Bed for Toddlers*. Play. Learn. Thrive. https://playlearnthrive.com/best-travel-bed-for-toddlers/

Gates, M. (n.d.-a). *Baby growth spurts*. BabyCenter. Retrieved August 17, 2023, from https://www.babycenter.com/baby/baby-development/baby-growth-spurts_40007276

Geddes, J. K. (2022, June 22). *How Do You Do the Pickup, Put Down Method of Sleep Training?* What to Expect. https://www.whattoexpect.com/first-year/sleep/pick-up-put-down-method-sleep-training/

Gettler, L. T., McKenna, J. J., McDade, T. W., Agustin, S. S., & Kuzawa, C. W. (2012). Does Co-sleeping Contribute to Lower Testosterone Levels in Fathers? Evidence from the Philippines. *PLoS ONE, 7*(9), e41559. https://doi.org/10.1371/journal.pone.0041559

Gold, T. (2017, July 20). *The 12 Hours by 12 Weeks Sleep Training Method - How to Implement It.* Huffington Post. https://www.huffpost.com/entry/the-12-hours-by-12-weeks-sleep-training-method-how_b_5970cee1e4b04dcf308d2aab

Iturmendi, A. (2018, December 7). *Dealing With Baby Jet Lag and Adjusting Fast To A New Time Zone.* ParentHood4Ever. https://www.parenthood4ever.com/baby-jet-lag-and-new-time-zone/

Jain, S. (2022). *How Often and How Much Should Your Baby Eat?* HealthyChildren.org. https://www.healthychildren.org/English/ages-stages/baby/feeding-nutrition/Pages/How-Often-and-How-Much-Should-Your-Baby-Eat.aspx

Kotlen, M. (2022). *How Much Breast Milk Should You Put in a Bottle for Your Baby?* Verywell Family. https://www.verywellfamily.com/how-much-breast-milk-should-i-put-in-a-bottle-431802

Kyte, J. (2018, November 24). *When Your Baby is Sick: How to Maintain a Sleep Routine.* Kyte Baby. https://kytebaby.com/blogs/news/when-your-baby-is-sick-how-to-maintain-a-sleep-routine

Lewis, J. (2023, June 21). *The strong bond between children and comfort objects.* Care for Kids. https://www.careforkids.com.au/blog/the-strong-bond-between-children-and-comfort-objects

LoMonaco, J. L. (2023, March 13). *How to support older siblings when your new baby is up all night.* Cradlewise. https://cradlewise.com/blog/how-to-support-older-siblings-when-your-new-baby-is-up-all-night

LoRe, A. (2023a). *Sleep training for 6 month olds and older babies: How to, methods and tips.* Huckleberry. https://huckleberrycare.com/blog/sleep-training-for-6-month-olds-and-older-babies

LoRe, A. (2023b, July 31). *Baby takes short naps: Why and how to extend short naps?* Huckleberry. https://huckleberrycare.com/blog/5-reasons-your-babys-naps-are-too-short

Marcin, A. (2020, June 24). *Cry It Out Method: Age, How Long Is Too Long, Possible Harm.* Healthline. https://www.healthline.com/health/baby/cry-it-out-method#what-it-is

Martinelli, K. (2023). *Finding a Sleep Training Method That Works for Your Family.* Child Mind Institute. https://childmind.org/article/choosing-a-sleep-training-method-that-works-for-your-family/

Mayo Clinic. (2022, November 24). *Postpartum Depression—Symptoms and Causes.* https://www.mayoclinic.org/diseases-conditions/postpartum-depression/symptoms-causes/syc-20376617

Mayo Clinic Staff. (2022, October 6). *Baby naps: Daytime sleep tips.* https://www.mayoclinic.org/healthy-lifestyle/infant-and-toddler-health/in-depth/baby-naps/art-20047421

McKenna, J. J. (2014). Night waking among breastfeeding mothers and infants: Conflict, congruence or both? *Evolution, Medicine, and Public Health, 2014*(1), 40–47. https://doi.org/10.1093/emph/eou006

Middlemiss, W., Granger, D. A., Goldberg, W. A., & Nathans, L. (2012). Asynchrony of mother–infant hypothalamic–pituitary–adrenal axis activity following extinction of infant crying responses induced during the transition to sleep. *Early Human Development, 88*(4), 227–232. https://doi.org/10.1016/j.earlhumdev.2011.08.010

Miller, S. G. (2017, February 27). *Here's How Much Less Sleep Women Get Once They Have Kids.* Live Science. https://www.livescience.com/58026-moms-get-less-sleep.html

Miller-Wilson, K. (2018, November 23). *Using Baby Night Lights*. LoveToKnow. https://www.lovetoknow.com/parenting/baby/baby-night-light

Mindell, J. A., Kuhn, B., Lewin, D. S., Meltzer, L. J., Sadeh, A., & American Academy of Sleep Medicine. (2006). Behavioral treatment of bedtime problems and night wakings in infants and young children. *Sleep, 29*(10), 1263–1276. https://pubmed.ncbi.nlm.nih.gov/17068979/

Mindell, J. A., Meltzer, L. J., Carskadon, M. A., & Chervin, R. D. (2009). Developmental aspects of sleep hygiene: Findings from the 2004 National Sleep Foundation Sleep in America Poll. *Sleep Medicine, 10*(7), 771–779. https://doi.org/10.1016/j.sleep.2008.07.016

Mindell, J. A., & Williamson, A. A. (2018). Benefits of a bedtime routine in young children: Sleep, development, and beyond. *Sleep Medicine Reviews, 40*(1), 93–108. https://doi.org/10.1016/j.smrv.2017.10.007

Mitchell, S. (n.d.). *8 Ways to Help Your Baby Sleep While Traveling*. Retrieved August 21, 2023, from https://www.helpingbabiessleep.com/blog/8-ways-help-baby-sleep-traveling

Mlynek, A. (2012, February 7). *The dos and don'ts of safe co-sleeping with your baby*. Today's Parent. https://www.todaysparent.com/baby/baby-sleep/the-debate-should-you-co-sleep/

Motroni, A. (2019, November 4). *The Pros and Cons of Baby-wise*. The Postpartum Party. https://thepostpartumparty.com/babywise/

The Mummy & Daddy Sleep Consultant. (2022, August 8). *Teething Symptoms & The Impact On Sleep*. https://themummyanddaddysleepconsultant.ie/teething-symptoms/

National Sleep Foundation. (2015). *Sleep Duration Recommendations*. https://www.paaap.org/uploads/1/2/4/3/124369935/551b74_0a25804f79b44994bb8db7ed9ed957db.pdf

Nemours KidsHealth. (2020). *Naps (for Parents)*. Kidshealth.org. https://kidshealth.org/en/parents/naps.html

Netmums. (2016, July 20). *Teaching your baby to sleep with (almost!) no tears*. https://www.netmums.com/baby/sleep-training-techniques---the-no-cry-approach

Noor-Mohammed, R., & Basha, S. (2012). Teething disturbances; prevalence of objective manifestations in children under age 4 months to 36 months. *Medicina Oral Patología Oral Y Cirugia Bucal, PMC3476083*, e491–e494. https://doi.org/10.4317/medoral.17487

*Nursery Lighting for Babies and Toddlers*. (2021, March 22). BlissLights. https://blisslights.com/blogs/blisslights/nursery-lighting-for-babies-and-toddlers

O'Connor, A. (2022, June 21). *Your Complete Guide to Baby Naps*. What to Expect. https://www.whattoexpect.com/first-year/child-sleep.aspx

O'Connor, A. (2023, January 31). *Is Your Baby Ready to Drop a Nap?* What to Expect. https://www.whattoexpect.com/first-year/ask-heidi/dropping-morning-nap.aspx

Office on Women's Health. (2017, January 31). *Pumping and storing breastmilk*. Womenshealth.gov. https://www.womenshealth.gov/breastfeeding/pumping-and-storing-breastmilk

Owens, J. (2020). *Behavioral sleep problems in children*. Up to date. https://www.uptodate.com/contents/behavioral-sleep-problems-in-children

Pacheco, D. (2021, June 9). *Sleep Deprivation and New Parenthood*. Sleep Foundation. https://www.sleepfoundation.org/sleep-deprivation/parents

Pacheco, D. (2023, April 26). *Infant Sleep Cycles: How Are They Different From Adults?* Sleep Foundation. https://www.sleepfoundation.org/baby-sleep/baby-sleep-cycle

Park, E. M., Meltzer-Brody, S., & Stickgold, R. (2013). Poor sleep maintenance and subjective sleep quality are associated with postpartum maternal depression symptom severity. *Archives of Women's Mental Health, 16*(6), 539–547. https://doi.org/10.1007/s00737-013-0356-9

Peacock, F. (2014, September 15). *How To Transition From Co-Sleeping To Solo Sleeping | 11 Helpful Tips*. BellyBelly. https://www.bellybelly.com.au/baby-sleep/transition-from-co-sleeping/

Primary Care Pediatrics at Nemours Children's Health. (n.d.). *Formula Feeding FAQs: How Much and How Often (for Parents)*. Kidshealth.org. https://kidshealth.org/en/parents/formulafeed-often.html

Quinn, G. E., Shin, C. H., Maguire, M. G., & Stone, R. A. (1999). Myopia and ambient lighting at night. *Nature, 399*(6732), 113–114. https://doi.org/10.1038/20094

Raising Children Network. (n.d.-a). *Babies: sleep*. https://raisingchildren.net.au/babies/sleep

Raising Children Network. (n.d.-b). *Baby sleep: 2-12 months*. https://raisingchildren.net.au/babies/sleep/understanding-sleep/sleep-2-12-months

Raising Children Network. (n.d.-c). *How to sleep better: 10 tips for children*. https://raisingchildren.net.au/toddlers/sleep/better-sleep-settling/sleep-better-tips

Raising Children Network. (2022). *Night weaning and phasing out night feeds: things to think about*. https://raisingchildren.net.au/babies/sleep/settling-routines/night-weaning

Raising Children Network. (2023a). *Introducing solids: why, when, what and how*. https://raisingchildren.net.au/babies/breastfeeding-bottle-feeding-solids/solids-drinks/introducing-solids

Raising Children Network. (2023b). *Moving from cot to bed*. https://raisingchildren.net.au/toddlers/sleep/where-your-child-sleeps/cot-to-bed

Richter, D., Krämer, M. D., Tang, N. K. Y., Montgomery-Downs, H. E., & Lemola, S. (2019). Long-term effects of pregnancy and childbirth on sleep satisfaction and duration of first-time and experienced mothers and fathers. *Sleep, 42*(4). https://doi.org/10.1093/sleep/zsz015

Rockwood, K. (2017). *The Best Baby Sleep Tips Ever*. Parents. https://www.parents.com/baby/sleep/tips/the-best-baby-sleep-tips-ever/

Romero, T. (2023, May 16). *Having a hard time falling back asleep at night? Don't watch the clock*. PhillyVoice. https://www.phillyvoice.com/how-fall-asleep-insomnia-clock-watching/

Ruggeri, A. (2022, February 9). *Should I Wake My Baby Up to Feed?* What to Expect. https://www.whattoexpect.com/first-year/ask-heidi/wake-to-feed.aspx

Santiago-Munoz, P. (2015, June 2). *Overcoming postpartum depression: Elaine's story | Your Pregnancy Matters*. UT Southwestern Medical Center. https://utswmed.org/medblog/overcoming-postpartum-depression/

Scatliffe, N., Casavant, S., Vittner, D., & Cong, X. (2019). Oxytocin and Early parent-infant interactions: a Systematic Review. *International Journal of Nursing Sciences*, 6(4), 445–453. https://doi.org/10.1016/j.ijnss.2019.09.009

Schuster, K., PsyD, Learning, is a neuropsychologist in the, Center, D., & Institute, D. of C. T. at the C. M. (2023). *Encouraging Good Sleep Habits*. Child Mind Institute. https://childmind.org/article/encouraging-good-sleep-habits/

*The Science behind baby sleep*. (n.d.). La Lune Consulting Pediatric Sleep Coach. Retrieved August 11, 2023, from https://www.laluneconsulting.com/blog/the-science-behind-baby-sleep

Sezici, E., & Yigit, D. (2017). Comparison between swinging and playing of white noise among colicky babies: A paired randomised controlled trial. *Journal of Clinical Nursing*, 27(3-4), 593–600. https://doi.org/10.1111/jocn.13928

Shaw, G. (2023). *Feeding Baby: How to Avoid Food Allergies*. WebMD. https://www.webmd.com/parenting/baby/introducing-new-foods

SickKids Staff. (2019). *About Kids Health*. Www.aboutkidshealth.ca. https://www.aboutkidshealth.ca/Article?contentid=710&language=English

Smith, J., & VanessaArbuthnott.co.uk. (2021, June 1). *Newborn Baby's Room: Why Light Control is Important*. HABA USA. https://www.habausa.com/blogs/blog-inspiration/newborn-babys-room-why-light-control-is-important

SnoozeShade. (n.d.). *Elizabeth Pantley—The No Cry Sleep Solution*. Retrieved August 17, 2023, from https://www.snoozeshade.com/pages/elizabeth-pantly-gentle-removal

Spencer, J. A., Moran, D. J., Lee, A., & Talbert, D. (1990). White noise and sleep induction. *Archives of Disease in Childhood*, 65(1), 135–137. https://doi.org/10.1136/adc.65.1.135

Stone, K. (2013, June 7). *Tips for Getting More Sleep & Protecting Your Milk Supply During PPD*. POSTPARTUM PROGRESS. https://postpartumprogress.com/tips-for-getting-more-sleep-protecting-your-milk-supply-during-ppd

Suni, E. (2020). *What is Circadian Rhythm?* (A. Dimitriu, Ed.). Sleep Foundation. https://www.sleepfoundation.org/circadian-rhythm

Swartz, J. (2012, November 28). *KidCo Inc. Recalls Children's PeaPod Travel Beds*. https://swartzlaw.com/kidco-inc-recalls-childrens-peapod-travel-beds/us

Taylor, M. (2022, November 22). *How to Stop Co-Sleeping With Your Baby or Toddler*. What to Expect. https://www.whattoexpect.com/toddler/sleep/how-to-stop-co-sleeping

Taylor, M. (2023, May 25). *Should You Try the Ferber Method on Your Baby?* What to Expect. https://www.whattoexpect.com/first-year/sleep/ferber-method-sleep-training/

*Teething: Tips for soothing sore gums*. (2018). Mayo Clinic. https://www.mayoclinic.org/healthy-lifestyle/infant-and-toddler-health/in-depth/teething/art-20046378

Tham, E., Schneider, N., & Broekman, B. (2017). Infant sleep and its relation with cognition and growth: a narrative review. *Nature and Science of Sleep, Volume 9*, 135–149. https://doi.org/10.2147/nss.s125992

*Tips for Nursery Lighting*. (2015, September 9). 1000Bulbs.com Blog. https://blog.1000bulbs.com/home/tips-for-nursery-lighting

Tracy Hogg Dies at 44. (n.d.). *Washington Post*. Retrieved August 16, 2023, from https://www.washingtonpost.com/archive/local/2004/12/07/tracy-hogg-dies-at-44/7923ca85-e73d-4845-94e8-aa9d29ff03c2/

University of Notre Dame. (n.d.). *NICU Standard 24: Ambient Lighting in Infant Care Areas*. NICU Recommended Standards. https://nicudesign.nd.edu/nicu-standards/nicu-standard-24-ambient-lighting-in-infant-care-areas/

West, K. (2015, January 21). *10 Reasons That Quality Sleep Matters For Your Baby*. The Sleep Lady. http://sleeplady.com/baby-sleep/10-reasons-that-quality-sleep-matters-for-your-baby/

Willes, N. (2017). *Getting your baby to sleep the baby sleep trainer way.*

Wood, S. (2023). *How to Sleep Train Your Baby (In Just 7 Days)*. Parents. https://www.parents.com/baby/sleep/issues/teach-your-baby-to-sleep-in-just-7-days/

Zwarensteyn, J. (2020, June 4). *How to Get Babies to Take Longer Naps - 8 Easy Tips for Day and Night*. Sleep Advisor. https://www.sleepadvisor.org/how-to-get-babies-to-nap-longer/